ARTHRITIS INTERRUPTED

Featuring The Arthritis Healing Diet

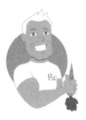

Jim Healthy Publications
P.O. Box 5699
Santa Fe, NM 87505

TABLE OF CONTENTS

INTRODUCTION

US DOCTORS HAVE HIT A BRICK WALL in the quest for an arthritis cure. If you're still suffering from either osteoarthritis (OA) or rheumatoid arthritis (RA), we're sure you noticed.

You're not alone. Nearly 50 million Americans are diagnosed with some form of arthritis – with millions more hobbling around not sure of the reason because they can't afford a doctor or medical care. Most often, OA is the cause.

Diagnosed or not, arthritis is the leading cause of disability in the US. And we're talking about 20% of the adult population, with that number expected to grow to nearly 70 million by 2030. Ten states are expected to see increases of 50% by then.

MODERN MEDICINE IS POWERLESS AGAINST IT

Sadly, even though arthritis is responsible for $128 billion of our total healthcare expenditure, patients are getting little in return for the money they are spending. Orthopedic specialists in this country have little to offer patients, with the exception of a few new drugs that control chronic RA inflammation.

OA patients have even fewer options. Conventional medical advice ranges from, "Well, that's aging for you!" … to reliance on anti-inflammatory drugs and COX-2 inhibitors (glorified aspirin that protects against gastric bleeding and ulcers) … or, ultimately, artificial joint replacement and/or various back surgeries.

"JUST LIVE WITH IT!"

Each one of these "solutions" carries some pretty serious health risks, medical dangers and nasty side effects…

Just recently, acetaminophen and anti-inflammatory drugs have been linked to even worse liver damage than previously thought. COX-2 arthritis medications have been long known to increase the chances of heart attack and stroke. And regular aspirin use is linked to stomach ulcers, gastrointestinal bleeding and vision problems.

Risks of joint replacement surgery risks the gamut from picking up a staph infection ... complications from anesthesia ... to recurring joint dislocation ... permanent muscle damage ... or lifetime disability (from "less than perfect" surgical outcomes that orthopedists try to keep from the public).

Another well-kept secret is that anti-inflammatory drugs and arthritis medications actually *accelerate* joint destruction – especially OA – because they inhibit the process by which the body usually repairs damaged cartilage and regenerates new joint tissue.

The only options from the US medical community to arthritis patients are, "Take these painkillers for now, and come back when your joints need replacing." Those aren't very satisfying choices.

THE HEALING POWER OF CERTAIN FOODS

But is this *truly* your only option? Absolutely not. Even though conventional orthopedists almost never mention them, there are plenty of arthritis healing foods, diet strategies, nutritional supplements and exercise routines plus *non-pharmaceutical* pain management techniques that can extend your joint comfort and functionality by extra years or decades – and allow you to postpone surgical intervention indefinitely.

These non-medical treatments for OA have real efficacy and plenty of scientific and clinical evidence behind them, as you'll see in these pages.

We wrote this book to fill a vital information gap. In the chapters ahead, you'll discover specific healing superfoods, medicinal herbs, nutritional supplements and other non-medical therapies which are well-documented to reduce pain and promote healing for both OA and RA.

WE'RE LIVING PROOF

The good news is that there is *plenty* you can do to control your arthritis (instead of *it* controlling you) without resorting to risky drugs and radical surgeries.

Both Jim and I are living proof. We're a pair of aging ex-jocks in our early 60s with a pile of excess miles on our joints and spines.

I'm an MD who wrestled in high school and college, and have been athletic all my life; downhill skiing was my passion for decades. Jim banged his bones and joints around football fields from pee-wee league to the semi-pros. He was a fierce martial artist for 15 years after that, and a basketball junkie until he was 50, when he took up the herky-jerky sport of tennis.

Our joints have gotten more than their fair share of wear and tear. Examine the x-rays of our knees and hips and it's hard to find very much cartilage. Yet we both live normal, active, pain-free (and drug-free!) lives thanks to The Arthritis Healing Diet™ and the many other arthritis-thwarting secrets we're about to share with you.

OUR 30-DAY ARTHRITIS HEALING PLAN

In this special e-book, we've combined our medical, health and nutritional knowledge to bring you literally hundreds of non-drug, non-surgical helpers and healers that can extend the mileage of your joints and spine … halt the progression of your arthritis … end your pain … increase your flexibility … and help you feel young again.

We've made it as simple as possible to benefit from these well-documented arthritis healing remedies without turning your schedule upside down or overwhelming you with "an entirely new lifestyle."

Our one-a-day approach adds one new arthritis healer to your life each day. How easy is that? Day-by-day, you'll be learning new ways to eat, move, control your pain, heal your joints—so you can begin to reverse your arthritis. At the end of our 30-day plan, you'll have your arthritis under control and feel like a new person! This simple, systematic approach frontloads the most powerful healers and therapeutic foods, so you'll experience the biggest benefits from Day One.

And because your diet is such an essential part of the healing process, we've included a number of original Arthritis Healing Recipes that feature the top arthritis super-healing foods that contain documented medicinal and anti-inflammatory properties. Not only are these meals especially healthful and healing for your joints, they're loaded with great flavor.

WHY YOU NEED A "MULTIPLE" APPROACH LIKE THIS

It would be nice if there were just one or two remedies that would fix your joints, but the human body is far too complex—and arthritis is far too stubborn.

In order to successfully "interrupt" arthritis, it needs to be addressed on a variety of fronts—molecular, nutritional, biochemical and physical—in order to halt its progression and coax its reversal.

Sadly, it's "not worth the effort" for the vast majority of arthritis patients. Either they don't believe such a simple, low-cost strategy can succeed where modern medicine has failed, or they aren't willing to make the lifestyle changes that can end their pain and restore their mobility.

This is a shame because the fun they're missing and the misery they're enduring (both unnecessarily, by the way) are probably making their life something to "get through" rather than a great gift to relish and enjoy. But that's not you, right?

DISCOVER YOUR POWER OVER ARTHRITIS

While there is still no cure for arthritis (and there may never be), our holistic plan is the next best thing. And it's never too early to get started on it because by age 40, 90% of the population has some osteoarthritic changes in their hips and/or knee joints that can be seen on x-rays. By age 75, virtually *everyone* has deterioration in at least one joint.

Very few people escape OA, but not everyone has to suffer from it. That's because the speed and severity at which the disease progresses is largely up to you. Here's why…

Generally, OA is slow-moving. Plenty of people have it for decades without experiencing any symptoms at all. Other people are hit with the sudden onset of pain and immobility as joints and/or spinal flexibility deteriorates quickly. What makes the difference? Three factors are at work in OA: genetics, your body's inflammation chemistry, and the environmental influences to which you're exposed.

Your individual DNA contains certain genes that determine your susceptibility to developing arthritis – and how fast or slow this happens. They do this, in part, by establishing the ratio of natural anti-inflammatory compounds (called "growth factors") in your joints to those responsible for inflammation (called *cytokines*). In other words, OA is fundamentally a molecular disease. It's *not* so much a result of physical wear and tear on your joints as it is the destructive effect of these caustic cytokines, mainly *interleukin-1* (IL-1) and *tumor necrosis factor-alpha* (TNF-a), which dissolve cartilage when joints are chronically inflamed. But, as you'll see, you have significant control over this destructive process.

Environmental factors play a very important role, too. These include injury and trauma to your joints … accumulated wear and tear … your body weight (which affects the load your joints carry) … physical activity and flexibility … ingested substances, including harmful medications, cigarette smoking and environmental toxins … and, perhaps most important of all, your diet.

While there isn't much you can do about the genes you inherited—although cutting-edge treatments now available in Europe are using biological compounds which boost the inflammation-fighting growth factors in a particular joint to stop pain, to halt OA's progression, and actually promote cartilage repair (see www.molecularorthopedia.com for details)—you definitely can alter your body's molecular chemistry through what you do and don't eat.

The day is near when rebuilding worn-out joint surfaces will be as easy as injecting stem cells into a joint to miraculously create a new layer of resilient cartilage. This is already happening in cutting-edge orthopedic clinics in Europe such as the Center for Molecular Orthopedics in Düsseldorf, Germany. Doctors there are also transplanting cartilage from a patient's own body or grown on miniature scaffolds in the lab. In addition, they are able to insert stem cell plugs that produce new cartilage, and/or small metal discs that encourage surrounding cartilage to overgrow them and repair worn spots. This new technology is amazing. Unfortunately, orthopedic advances in the US lag far behind, mostly due to our medical politics.

The good news is that you don't have to wait for our medical system to change. There is plenty you can do right now to halt your arthritis in its tracks and reverse its direction without needing a doctor's assistance. You hold the key to your own healing and it rests in…

THE SECRET TO CONTROLLING INFLAMMATION

Arthritis is primarily a disease of inflammation, which also holds true for most medical conditions. What you eat is critical to your health and healing. By eating more foods that exert a significant anti-inflammatory effect in your body, you can minimize your joint pain, while increasing your comfort and mobility. And because inflammation destroys joint cartilage, you'll also be slowing the progression of your disease.

Continuing to eat pro-inflammatory foods will make your pain worse. These foods and other substances can trigger inflammation flare-ups, increase the amount of cartilage-destroying enzymes in your joints, irritate nerve endings to make pain worse and accelerate the progression of your disease.

WHICH OUTCOME DO YOU WANT?

Perhaps no disease makes you feel "old before your time" like arthritis. Instead of popping out of bed and hitting the ground running, you drag yourself through the morning, waiting for your joints to "warm up." You turn your entire torso to see something behind you, instead of merely rotating your neck on its axis. You limp. You hobble. You ache. You hurt. You probably don't bend or run or dance or frolic like you used to. And your movements may have slowed down to a snail's pace. These are the hallmarks of being "old."

Furthermore, reduced physical activity has negative effects on cardiovascular health, brain function, weight gain and every organ in the human body. We were born to move – and our body works best when we stay in motion. To stop moving is to begin dying. Some immobility comes naturally with aging. But much of it is avoidable – and even *reversible*. The secret is minimizing the inflammation in your joints, vertebrae, and elsewhere. That's exactly what The Arthritis Healing Diet™ can do for you. So let's get going…

Stephen Sinatra, MD
Jim Healthy

P.S. – Please tell us your story! We'd love to hear how you are "interrupting" your arthritis. Send your personal story to jimhealthy@arthrtisinterrupted.com, and, with your permission, we'll publish it to inspire and motivate others. Photos are welcome, too.

(+)

DAY 1: SWITCH TO DRUG-FREE PAIN RELIEVERS

HEALER: **Stop the pain and inflammation in your joints with these non-drug analgesics and anti-inflammatory remedies. They work just as well as pharmaceuticals, but are far safer – and better for your joints.**

THE VERY FIRST STEP in healing your arthritis is having the ability to stop your pain if and when it arises. But providing relief must <u>not</u> come at the expense of causing more damage to your joints and hastening their destruction, or endangering your heart, liver, kidneys or other organs.

HELP – DON'T HURT – YOUR JOINTS' CHANCES OF REAL HEALING

To give your joints every chance of healing, think of yourself as a skillful fireman. Use water, not gasoline (see The Trouble with Painkillers and Arthritis Drugs, beginning on page 16), to extinguish the "fire" in them. This will minimize the damage you do when snuffing out your pain.

Once you discover which of these non-drug alternatives work best for you if/when pain and inflammation strike, you can focus your energy on the healing and rebuilding process. Our long-term strategy is for you to feed your system as many anti-inflammatory foods and compounds as you can in order to prevent painful flare-ups. But in the short-term, you're going to need "911 pain relief" that won't endanger your health or make your arthritis worse. Since everyone responds differently to medications and nutrients, we suggest you experiment until you find one of these no-drug pain relievers that satisfies you. Here are the best of the bunch, from our experience and research....

7

FOR FAST-ACTING PAIN RELIEF

▶**White willow: the original aspirin.** White willow bark (*Salix spp.*) is an ancient pain-reliever that has been used for centuries. It contains *salicin*, a natural analgesic compound. In 1897, the Bayer Company in Germany synthesized salicin into *acetylsalicylic acid* and marketed the first aspirin, which went on to become the bestselling drug in history. But aspirin carries some serious dangers and side effects, not the least of which are ulcers and bleeding in the stomach and GI tract. White willow is a very effective pain-reliever and produces no uncomfortable side effects (although people with peptic ulcers or gastritis are advised against using it). Use it as you would aspirin or any NSAID (*non-steroidal anti-inflammatory drug*), but follow the directions on the label. White willow is widely available in capsule, tablet or tincture form.

▶**Let devil's claw scratch your backache.** Devil's Claw (*Harpagophytum procumbens*) is a good choice when OA attacks your spine, causing chronic back pain. It contains well-documented analgesic and anti-inflammatory compounds. Devil's claw is widely used in Europe where it is officially approved for treating pain and inflammation by Commission E, the German counterpart of our FDA. In a six-week head-to-head study at the University of Freiburg, Germany, devil's claw outperformed the arthritis drug Vioxx in relieving back pain by 50%—without the drug's side effects. Several studies also confirm that devil's claw relieves the aches, pain and stiffness of OA, the most common form of joint pain. French researchers showed that it works just as well as a nonsteroidal anti-inflammatory drug (NSAID) in reducing painful OA of the knee or hip, and is much safer. Unlike NSAIDs, devil's claw doesn't interfere with blood clotting, making it safe for those taking blood-thinning drugs. Check with your doctor first.

▶**Put out the fire with chili pepper cream.** The compound that gives chili peppers its "hotness"—*capsaicin*—temporarily desensitizes nerve receptors that register pain. It's like cutting the line of communication from your sore joints to your brain. Some studies show that arthritis patients are able to cut their pain intensity in half after using a topical capsaicin cream. Capsaicin ointments and creams are sold in pharmacies and health stores. Shop for a 0.075% capsaicin cream and rub it on painful joints one to four times daily. You'll get the best results when you use it for an arthritis flare-up, rather than to control everyday pain and stiffness.

► **Boswellia: Mother Nature's Celebrex®.** Derived from the bark of India's *Boswellia serrata* tree, this herb can relieve OA symptoms quite quickly, and it's much safer than aspirin. A 2008 study run by the University of California at Davis confirms that boswellia extract is safe enough for long-term use—with no apparent side-effects. This comes as no surprise, given that traditional Indian Ayurvedic physicians have relied on it for centuries for its anti-inflammatory properties. Recent studies involving RA patients found that the vast majority experienced less inflammation and stiffness within two to four weeks of using boswellia.

In a study published in the journal *Arthritis Research & Therapy*, researchers gave boswellia extract to a group of people with OA with classic symptoms including pain, stiffness, and limited movement. But after taking the extract for just one week, their symptoms were relieved.

Another study showed boswellia to be effective for knee OA. After taking 333 mg daily, patients reported less knee pain and more mobility, and they were able to walk farther than those who didn't get the pain-relieving herb.

How it works: boswellia limits inflammation by stopping *leukotriene synthesis*, which initiates the inflammation cycle. It works for the symptoms of both RA and OA, and can be applied directly to the skin over the joints as a cream, or taken in pill form.

Look for products containing 60% *boswellic acids*, the plant's active ingredient, and take 300-400 mg by mouth three times daily. Or you can use the cream for as long as you need, rubbing a popcorn-sized dab into the skin over your aching joint every four to six hours. If you're pregnant or immune-compromised, check with your doctor first.

FOR LONG-TERM PAIN PREVENTION

Staying a giant step ahead of inflammation and the painful stiffness it causes will smooth out the usual rollercoaster ride of "good and bad days" that those of us with arthritis know all too well. You could never accomplish this safely with drugs, but certain supplements (and many foods, as you'll soon see) can keep your bloodstream well supplied with enough inflammation-squelching and pain-blocking compounds so that those arthritic hills and valleys turn into a smooth highway. Experiment with these proven pain-preventers until you discover your favorite...

▶**SAM-e provides relief in just 7 days.** When University of California at Irvine researchers tested *S-adenosyl-L-methionine* (no wonder it's name is shortened to SAM-e) head-to-head against the COX-2 arthritis drug Celebrex, they found it reduced pain and improved joint function as well as the pricey pharmaceutical. But European doctors weren't surprised. They've been using SAM-e to treat people with OA and RA for years.

In fact, when researchers conducted a meta-analysis (a comparison of many studies) on SAM-e, 11 clinical trials confirmed that the supplement was as effective as ibuprofen and other anti-inflammatory drugs at reducing pain and boosting mobility –with none of the drugs' side effects.

SAM-e is a chemical that already exists in our bodies. Taking a bit more as a supplement has been shown to produce painkilling and anti-inflammatory effects in as little as seven days. This is one valuable supplement!

But please "B" aware: you need healthy levels of the B vitamins in your bloodstream for SAM-e to do its work, so take a B-complex 100 every day along with your daily 1,200 mg of SAM-e, the amount used in the U of C study.

You may find yourself smiling more, too. Many people take SAM-e to relieve depression, at a dose of 1,600 mg daily. Research shows it increases the feel-good brain chemicals serotonin and dopamine. Check with your doctor to be sure you aren't risking any potential interactions with drugs such as antidepressants and MAO inhibitors.

Another tip: inspect the packaging before buying to be sure the product carries a USP or GMP quality seal, bears a reasonable expiration date and comes in foil blister-packs (SAM-e degrades rapidly when exposed to direct light).

▶**MSM relieves arthritis pain by 80%.** Studies reveal that most people with arthritis are deficient in naturally-occurring sulfur compounds which the body needs to maintain strong connective tissue and mediate nerve impulses that transmit pain. Being deficient in sulfur also means your body isn't regenerating cartilage effectively.

Methylsulfonylmethane (MSM for short) is a potent sulfur compound found in vegetables, fruits, meats and grains. It's also available in higher concentrations as a supplement.

How MSM relieves pain: researchers at the UCLA School of Medicine found that OA patients who took MSM for six weeks experienced a whopping 80% reduction in their pain. That level of pain relief rivals strong pharmaceutical painkillers—but without their side effects.

MSM improves joint function, too. The Arthritis Foundation reports that a pilot study in 2006 showed that 6,000 mg of MSM daily boosted physical function and reduced pain, with nary a side effect. To give it a try, start with 3,000 mg daily, taking MSM with food, and build up to 5,000 mg per day. You can take as much as 10 grams if you need to. By starting slowly and taking MSM with food, you'll be able to get a handle on any mild GI side effects. If you're taking a blood-thinner, ask your doctor's permission before trying MSM.

▶ **ASU: the new arthritis healer on the block.** This promising new arthritis supplement is a mouthful to pronounce—*avocado soybean unsaponifiables* (ASU)—but swallowing 300 mg daily may be worth the trouble if you have arthritis. Research published in the *Journal of Rheumatology* demonstrates that ASU encourages cartilage repair and slows its destruction.

Four well-done studies found that taking the ASU tablets eases stiffness and pain in hips and knees, and can help patients reduce their intake of NSAIDs such as ibuprofen and naproxen. In two of the studies, patients received so much relief after just three months that they were able to cut back on NSAID pain-relievers. Scientists believe ASU improves arthritis symptoms by inhibiting the body's production of inflammatory chemicals.

But more isn't always better. Researchers found that taking more than 300 mg of ASU daily doesn't confer any additional benefits. They also say it can take up to eight weeks to start feeling ASU's effects, so be patient. You'll get continued symptom relief for up to eight weeks should you discontinue taking the supplement.

What about safety? French researchers have checked and ASU has passed with flying colors. Because it's available only by prescription there, the French government has evaluated its record for more than 15 years and found no problems.

While avocado and soy are healthful foods, eating massive quantities won't give you the benefits of ASU oils because they need to be extracted from the soy and avocado fibers before our joints can utilize them. The ASUs are too tightly bound to the plant fiber to be readily available to the human body.

▶ **Pycnogenol: the bark that stops OA's bite.** Otherwise known as French maritime pine bark extract, pycnogenol eases joint pain and stiffness, but without side effects. Studied in over 200 clinical trials, it has proven itself effective under the tightest scrutiny. In two recent trials, OA patients who took pycnogenol for three months saw their joint pain and stiffness diminish by up to 55%. As a result, they required fewer pain-relieving drugs such as NSAIDs and COX-2 inhibitors. Relief resulted from pycnogenol's extraordinary antioxidant and anti-inflammatory properties.

Bonus: pycnogenol lowers LDL and raises HDL (good) cholesterol to protect against heart disease. It also reduces blood pressure and the risk of blood clots, two other serious risks for possible heart attack. Furthermore, it's been shown to help control blood sugar in people with Type 2 diabetes. It also can ease menstrual pain, allowing women to cut in half the days they took pain meds. Last but not least, a new study shows it helps prevent jet lag.

For best results, take a 50 mg tablet two or three times daily with food – but don't surpass 200 mg a day. Check with your doctor first, especially if you're on any hypertension medication.

▶ **Bromelain: the pain-blocker in pineapple.** Bromelain is a protein-dissolving enzyme found in the pineapple plant. It possesses well-documented inflammation-fighting powers. Researchers have found that bromelain works like heavy-duty anti-inflammatory pharmaceutical drugs, but without the side effects. The University Of Maryland Medical Center reports that bromelain may help cut the pain of RA. It also seems to be as effective as a NSAID (like ibuprofen) against OA pain.

How it works: when bromelain reaches your bloodstream, its *proteolytic enzymes* consume the protein gunk that causes inflammation, while simultaneously driving down your body's production of joint-inflaming chemicals.

Be sure to take bromelain on an empty stomach though, so that the enzymes don't digest your meal instead of the inflammation-causing debris. Take from 500 mg to 2,000 mg daily, between meals.

(-)

DAY 2: BACK OFF OF PAINKILLERS

HURTER: **Cut back until you completely discontinue the use of pain relievers, anti-inflammatory drugs (NSAIDs), acetaminophen and COX-2 arthritis medications. Here's why...**

WHEN YOU'RE HURTING, it's natural to want relief. But if you have OA and turn to a conventional pain-reliever, that temporary comfort comes with a big price tag. All of these drugs carry their own set of health risks, dangers and side effects. In addition, even though they relieve your symptoms, studies show they actually accelerate the progression of OA by inhibiting the synthesis of *proteoglycans*, which are the molecules that attract water to cartilage so it stays moist and plump.

But halting inflammation as quickly as possible is necessary to avoid the destructive effects of chronic inflammation. So if you have a sudden flare-up from an injury or strenuous activity and exhaustion, by all means take an anti-inflammatory immediately to halt it.

Long-term use, on the other hand, is ill advised. You may feel better, but beneath the surface these drugs can be causing serious health problems – and perhaps even risking your life. Let's examine the risks of each...

THE PROBLEMS WITH PAINKILLERS AND ARTHRITIS DRUGS

In June, 2009, an advisory committee recommended that the FDA place new restrictions on products containing acetaminophen, one of the nation's bestselling pain-relieving agents. New studies have emerged revealing an even greater risk of toxicity, liver failure and death.

Acetaminophen is sold over-the-counter under the brand names Tylenol®, "aspirin-free" Anacin®, Excedrin®, Datril®, Liquiprin® and as an ingredient in numerous cold medicines. It is also present in many prescription drugs, which combine acetaminophen with narcotics. Billions of doses of these pain-relieving drugs are prescribed annually, including Vicodin, Lortab, Maxidone, Norco, Zydone, Tylenol with codeine, Percocet, Endocet, and Darvocet.

According to studies done between 1990 and 1998, acetaminophen-related overdoses cause 56,000 emergency room visits, 26,000 hospitalizations and 458 deaths annually. Those reported figures may actually be much higher.

The panel of doctors is now advising that a single adult dose of acetaminophen should be no more than 650 mg, significantly less than the current 1,000 mg contained in two tablets of many over-the-counter pain products. It also recommended decreasing the maximum total dose for the span of 24 hours, which is currently at 4,000 mg.

These new dangers are added to those already recognized, which include irritation to the stomach lining with occasional use, and bleeding ulcers in those taking a daily dose of 2,000 mg or more. This surprised many physicians because acetaminophen was thought to be easier on the stomach than aspirin and other NSAIDs.

THE DANGERS OF NSAIDS

NSAIDs (short for nonsteroidal anti-inflammatory drugs) are either prescribed or recommended when inflammation accompanies pain. The three types of NSAIDs are salicylates (such as aspirin), traditional NSAIDs (see list below) and COX-2 selective inhibitors.

The Most Common NSAIDs Used for Arthritis:

- Ansaid (generic name flurbiprofen)
- Arthrotec (generic name diclofenac with misoprostol)
- Aspirin (acetylated / non-acetlyted salicylates)
- Cataflam (generic name diclofenac potassium)
- Celebrex (generic name celecoxib)
- Clinoril (generic name sulindac)
- Daypro (generic name oxaprozin)
- Disalcid (generic name salsalate)

- Dolobid (generic name diflunisal)
- Feldene (generic name piroxicam)
- Ibuprofen (brand names include Motrin, Advil, Mediprin, Nuprin, Motrin IB)
- Indocin (generic name indomethacin)
- Ketoprofen (brands names include Orudis, Oruvail, Actron, Orudis KT)
- Lodine (generic name etodolac)
- Meclomen (generic name meclofenamate sodium)
- Mobic (generic name meloxicam)
- Nalfon (generic name fenoprofen)
- Naproxen (brand names include Naprosyn, Aleve, Naprelan, Anaprox)
- Ponstel (generic name mefanamic acid)
- Relafen (generic name nabumetone)
- Tolectin (generic name tolmetin sodium)
- Trilisate (generic name choline magnesium trisalicylate)
- Voltaren (generic name diclofenac sodium)

HOW NSAIDS WORK

NSAIDs halt inflammation by inhibiting the enzyme *cyclooxygenase* (known as COX), which transforms arachidonic acid into prostaglandins and leukotrienes. This draws plasma fluid and extra white blood cells into the joint as the first stage of healing.

Prostaglandins are hormone-like agents that regulate pain and the inflammation response. But prostaglandins serve other functions as well, such as protecting the stomach lining, promoting clotting of the blood and maintaining blood flow to the kidneys when their function is reduced. By blocking the entire COX enzyme, NSAIDs decrease the protective roles that prostaglandins play. This is how NSAIDs cause stomach irritation and bleeding, fluid retention and decreased kidney function. Fluid retention also can cause elevated blood pressure, which leads to a greater risk of heart problems, stroke and kidney disease.

The longer you take NSAIDs – and the higher the dose – the more likely you are to suffer serious side effects and damage.

- Continuous use of NSAIDs can result in kidney failure and liver disease, plus stomach ulcers and bleeding.

- NSAIDs (particularly indomethacin) can interfere with anti-hypertension medications and can cause cardiac failure in patients who take beta-blockers, angiotensin-converting enzyme (ACE) inhibitors or diuretics.

■ As previously mentioned, long-term use of NSAIDs has been shown to have a damaging effect on chondrocyte (cartilage cells) function, making arthritis worse.

THE COX-2 ARTHRITIS DRUGS

In response to these dangers, drug chemists created the COX-2 selective inhibitors.

It helps to understand that there are two forms of the COX enzyme, referred to as COX-1 and COX-2, and NSAIDs block both. COX-1 is the protective form, while COX-2 is involved in the inflammation pathway.

Popular COX-2 Inhibitor Drugs:

■ Celebrex (Celecoxib)
■ Licofelone (Dual COX/LOX)
■ Prexige (Lumiracoxib)
■ Vioxx (Rofecoxib – now off the market due to increased incidence of heart attacks)
■ Arcoxia (Etoricoxib)
■ Bextra (Valdecoxib)

By blocking only the COX-2 without interfering with the protective effects of COX-1, scientists hoped these new drugs would be a major breakthrough in safe pain management. But results have been disappointing.

One problem has been that the pain relief they produce is equal to or less than NSAIDs. Another is that the incidence of stomach ulcers is about the same. More troubling is their link to higher rates of heart attack and other coronary problems. A study involving 375,000 adults showed that taking Vioxx for more than five days produced a 70% higher risk of heart disease. An earlier study revealed a 400% higher incidence of heart attacks compared to arthritis patients who took a common NSAID. These and other findings led to Vioxx being withdrawn from the market in 2005.

But serious doubts still persist about safety and efficacy of the remaining COX-2 drugs. Not the least of these concerns is that they may impair the ability of cartilage to repair itself. How ironic that an FDA-approved drug for the treatment of OA may actually worsen the condition. That's not the result you want, is it? So promise your joints that you'll never again resort to these conventional drugs. It's the first step toward their true healing.

A FEW WORDS ABOUT CORTISONE

Cortisone injections are often presented as a solution for joint pain and limited mobility. But you should think twice before agreeing to them. Here's why…

While cortisone can provide short-term relief from unbearable inflammation and pain, this reprieve is only temporary—and carries some problems with it. Because it's a steroid, cortisone works by suppressing your immune system to block its normal response to inflammation. With the body's warning system (pain, discomfort and immobility) shut down, it's easy to damage the joint further without feeling or knowing it. This can cause a buildup of adhesions, scar tissue, bone spurs and further loss of cartilage, leaving surgery and/or joint replacement as the only options. Cortisone also causes deterioration of cartilage, connective tissue and bone, which is why most doctors usually limit a patient to no more than two injections per year at six month intervals. But there is a more serious danger in cortisone therapy…

Since it depresses the immune system, cortisone can also leave you vulnerable to cancer and various infections. Each of us has cancer cells and viruses in our body at all times, but they are kept in check by our immune system. Long before a cancer is detected, it usually has been present in the body for years (or decades) in a suppressed state thanks to our immune cells. Suppressing or weakening the immune system can upset this balance, triggering an outbreak of a pathological virus or cancer proliferation. This is particularly dangerous if you've had cancer before and are currently in remission. It's well known that dormant tumors can suddenly re-activate during times of stress because it weakens immunity. Cortisone can have the same consequence and isn't worth the risk.

(+)

DAY 3: GET HOOKED ON FISH OIL

HEALER: Begin taking 1,000 mg (usually one capsule) of high-quality omega-3 fish oil or krill oil three times per day.

OPTION 1: If you are already doing this, you can increase your dose to 3,000 mg three times per day for maximum benefit.

THE FASTEST, EASIEST WAY to control recurring joint pain and inflammation while improving the health of your joints is by taking omega-3 fish oil capsules. That's why it's considered the world's #1 arthritis supplement. Here's why…

HOW FISH OIL CONTROLS ARTHRITIS PAIN

Inflammation is responsible for that tight, aching sensation in your knees, hips, shoulders, hands and spine. But instead of reaching for the ibuprofen for pain relief, you can get a similar degree of comfort from a few capsules of fish oil. They contain omega-3 fatty acids, a super-healing polyunsaturated fat that produces a natural anti-inflammatory effect, offering the same relief as aspirin and other NSAID drugs, but without the health risks or adverse side effects.

MOTHER NATURE'S INFLAMMATION-FIGHTER

Studies show that people with moderate joint deterioration due to OA or RA experience less pain when they control the inflammation in their joints and in the body as a whole. And research clearly demonstrates the remarkable capacity of fish oil to ease inflammation and pain in people with arthritis.

Studies also show that consuming omega-3s stimulates the body's own production of *resolvins*, natural compounds which calm joint soreness and pain. Resolvins are fats manufactured from *eicosapentaenoic acid* (EPA) and *docosahexaenoic acid* (DHA) found in high-quality omega-3 fish oil.

FOR LONG-TERM PAIN RELIEF

The ability of omega-3 fish oil to ease inflammation and the pain of arthritis is well-documented. Studies show that people with OA and RA who take fish oil experience a significant reduction in joint inflammation almost immediately. More importantly, fish oil reduces arthritis pain by at least 50%, and sometimes more. That kind of relief is on a par with the top anti-inflammatory drugs.

In fact, fish oil capsules are so powerful, studies show they allow arthritis patients to quit their COX-2 arthritis medications and other anti-inflammatory NSAID drugs. Other research demonstrates that the anti-inflammatory effects of fish oil are almost identical to aspirin and other pain-relieving drugs such as ibuprofen and naproxen, but without the side effects. And a 2005 study noted even better effects for people with RA when olive oil was included in their diet. (More about this on Day 12.)

People with OA and RA who consume omega-3 fish regularly experience less inflammation and pain, with studies showing an immediate and significant reduction in joint inflammation. In one notable trial, patients who took daily fish oil capsules (the equivalent of a nightly salmon dinner or lunchtime can of sardines) for 14 weeks reduced their joint tenderness and pain by a full 50% compared to those who didn't get any fish oil. And those benefits lasted for as long as a month after the fish oil was stopped.

A HEALING FAT LIKE NO OTHER

So profound is omega-3s' anti-inflammatory power that it is beneficial in the treatment and prevention of a variety of medical conditions, including cardiovascular disease, high cholesterol, high blood pressure, diabetes, cancer, osteoporosis, inflammatory bowel disease (IBD), asthma, macular degeneration, PMS and others. Symptoms of omega-3 deficiency include extreme tiredness (fatigue), poor memory, dry skin, heart problems, mood swings or depression and poor circulation.

DO FISH OIL CAPSULES CONTAIN MERCURY?

What about the reported mercury contamination of fish? Does this mean fish oil is also dangerous? No. Researchers at Consumer Labs (www.consumerlabs.com) evaluated 20 different brands and found no detectable mercury levels. Almost all fish oil companies thoroughly filter their products to remove mercury residues.

CHECK LABELS TO BE SURE

Only purchase fish oil supplements labeled as having undergone *molecular distillation*, a process that eliminates toxins. And be sure the product you pick contains a minimum a minimum of 500 mg EPA and DHA combined.

THE HEALING DOSE

For maximum benefit, people with arthritis should take one to three 1000-mg capsules three times daily. When shopping, look for a supplement with at least 500 mg of omega-3 per dose – in the ideal ratio of 3:2 (300 mg of DHA to 200 mg of EPA). A word of caution: fish oil can thin your blood. So if you're taking a blood-thinning drug like *warfarin* (Coumadin) or *clopedigrel* (Plavix), talk to your doctor first if you take more than 2 grams daily.

If you're on blood sugar-lowering medications, taking omega-3s may increase your fasting blood sugar levels. Use them with caution if you're on blood sugar-lowering medications, such as *glipizide* (Glucotrol and Glucotrol XL), *glyburide* (Micronase or Diabeta), *glucophage* (Metformin), or insulin. Omega-3 supplements may increase your need for these medications, so be sure to consult your doctor first.

OTHER OMEGA-3 OPTIONS

Sea creatures aren't the sole source of omega-3s. Another component of omega-3 is *alpha-linolenic acid* (ALA), which is found in flaxseed oil. Your body converts a portion of ALA into EPA and DHA. ALA is also found in pumpkin seed oil, perilla seed and walnut oil. (More about these non-fish sources of omega-3s in the days ahead.)

HANDLE WITH CARE

Fish oil, krill oil and flaxseed oil should be kept refrigerated, or else their delicate omega-3 fats will become oxidized and rancid. Ingesting oxidized oils and fats is like pouring free radical molecules into your body. This can have dreadful consequences for your joints, plus it can trigger artery plaque formation, accelerated aging, and generalized inflammation.

(-)

DAY 4: CUT BACK ON OMEGA-6 FOODS

HURTER: **Start cutting back on foods which are high in omega-6 fatty acids. Not only do they trigger the inflammation response in your body, but they diminish your body's reserves of beneficial omega-3s.**

IMAGINE SOMEONE GAVE YOU a bottle of pills labeled "Arthritis Pain Activator" and that every time you took two, your arthritis would flare-up so viciously that you could hardly bear it. You'd have to be crazy to "take two every four hours" if the label advised you to, wouldn't you?

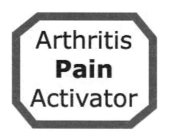

Generally speaking, that's the effect certain foods and substances can produce in your joints. And some of the most troublesome pain-provokers are foods containing excessive amounts of omega-6 fatty acids.

WHY OMEGA-6 FOODS ARE BAD FOR ARTHRITIS

Omega-6s and omega-3s are essential fatty acids, and both are important to good health. (They're called "essential" because your body can't produce them, so you must come from your diet). But here's a crucial distinction to remember if you have arthritis: too many omega-6s in your diet tend to cause inflammation, while omega-3s calm it down.

It's not that omega-6s are inherently evil (remember, they're "essential" to your health.), but when they're out of balance with omega-3s, the body churns out hormone-like substances called *eicosanoids*, which are highly inflammatory.

Thousands of years ago when humans ate foods in their natural forms, our diet consisted of two parts omega-6s to one part omega-3s (2:1). That's the ideal balance for optimal health and for minimal inflammation. Today, the ratio is closer to 20:1 in our modern diet.

Many scientists believe this overwhelmingly out-of-balance amount of omega-6s in our diet today is one of the main reasons for the dramatic increase in inflammation-driven medical conditions such as diabetes, heart disease, Alzheimer's and our old nemesis, arthritis. So to minimize arthritis pain and stiffness, choose foods rich in anti-inflammatory omega-3s, while limiting your intake of those containing a lot of omega-6s.

WHICH FOODS ARE HIGHEST IN OMEGA-6S?

Most omega-6s in our modern diet comes from refined wheat products and cheap, vegetable-based polyunsaturated oils (PUFAs), including corn, soybean, cottonseed, safflower, sunflower and canola. Corn and soybean oil contain 50% omega-6 and almost no omega-3. While canola oil contains 20% omega-6 to 10% omega-3, this amount isn't significant. It also oxidizes readily in the bloodstream and encourages free radical damage which is directly linked to inflammation. (You'll read more about this danger in the days ahead.)

THE TOP 10 OMEGA-6 FOODS

Locate the foods below in your own pantry or fridge and tape one of the "arthritis pain activator" labels (see p. 31) on them to remind yourself of the consequences that can occur from eating them....

1. Refined, polyunsaturated vegetables oils (canola, safflower, sunflower, corn)
2. Microwave popcorn with butter "flavoring"
3. All fast foods, especially the deep-fried ones
4. Most commercial salad dressings and dips
5. Granola bars and most energy bars
6. Processed snacks, including chips and crackers

7. Baked goods, such as coffee-cakes and cookies
8. Mayonnaise
9. Veggie burgers
10. Tub margarines

BALANCE YOUR OMEGAS FOR HEALTHIER, HAPPIER JOINTS

Your joints will feel much better if you eat fewer items on the list above. And be sure to add more fresh fruits, vegetables, omega-3 fish, lean meats, lentils, beans and whole grains to your diet because these are the foundation of The Arthritis Healing Diet™. These whole foods should comprise at least 80% or more of your day's nutrition. Snack on nuts and seeds, too. They contain omega-6s in their healthful original form, as do high-quality meats. Remember: it's easier and smarter to add more good foods to your diet than to fight your cravings for the bad ones.

Bring your total omegas into balance by consuming more omega-3s foods such as ground flaxseed, walnuts, cold-water fish and omega-3 fortified eggs. To get the maximum healing benefit of omega-3s, the fish oil supplements you're already taking will be a help. Your joints will thank you.

For optimal health and joint comfort, cook with small quantities of high-quality, natural oils such as coconut and sesame oils. Use extra virgin olive oil for dressing salads and veggies – as you'll see on Day 12, it's the most anti-inflammatory oil of them all.

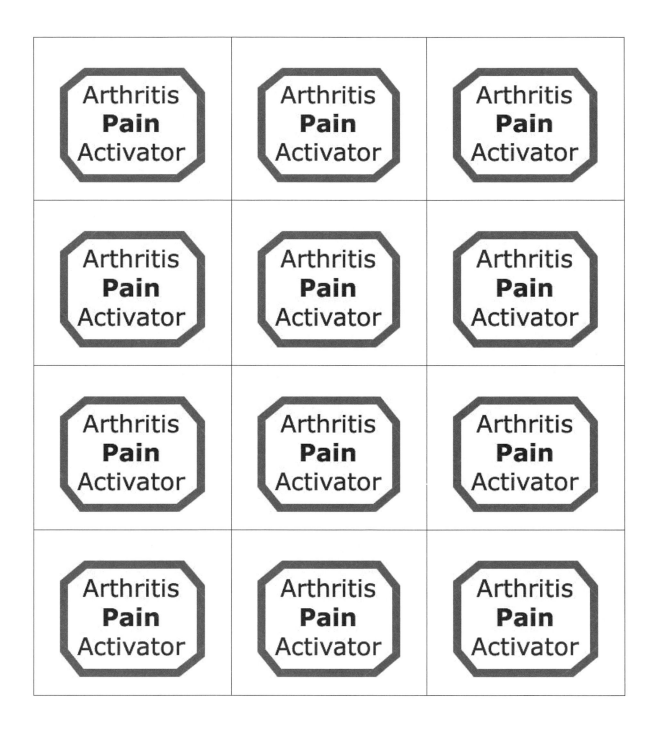

(+)

DAY 5: ARTHRITIS-HEALING BEVERAGES

HEALER: **These beverages contain powerful anti-inflammatory agents and antioxidant vitamins that protect and heal your joints…**

SINCE CARTILAGE IS 80% WATER, it's important to stay hydrated throughout the day. But why drink ordinary water when you can sip on beverages that discourage—and even reverse —inflammation, while actually healing your joints? Here are our favorites…

"PAIN-FREE" GREEN TEA

Green tea is at least 5,000 years old, but its healing benefits are knocking the socks off of modern-day arthritis researchers. For one thing, green tea is abundant in an antioxidant called *epigalloatechin-3-gallate* (EGCG) which has 20 times the power of vitamin C, making it one of the top defenders against free radical damage.[1]

More importantly, solid evidence shows that green tea's natural compounds block inflammatory cytokines (harmful enzyme-like agents), which destroy cartilage in arthritic joints when they are chronically inflamed. The usually conservative Arthritis Foundation was so impressed by this research that it named green tea as one of the top "10 Supplements Worth Considering" for alleviating the symptoms of RA and OA.

---

[1] **Free radicals** are destructive molecules produced by normal oxidation, be it from normal respiration (breathing) or when our bodies transform food into energy. One visible example of free radicals at work is when a slice of fresh apple turns brown when exposed to air. Free radical molecules lack one electron, which drives them to steal an electron from healthy oxygen molecules. This process damages healthy cells and tissues, while creating new generations of free radicals. The accumulation of excess free radicals in the body is thought to be responsible for the aging process and the degeneration of healthy tissue, including joint cartilage.

Dozens of studies have found that drinking tea reduces inflammation, slows the breakdown of cartilage and may even help prevent arthritis in the first place. You get all these benefits without any of the adverse side effects that drugs can pose. And green tea has a healing and preventative effect on many other medical conditions, including memory problems, heart disease and diabetes, just to name a few.

If you're accustomed to drinking coffee throughout the day, try making your first warm beverage of the morning a cup of green tea. It's faster and easier than brewing a pot of coffee and it packs nearly the same caffeine kick. Work toward replacing some of the coffee you normally drink with green tea for the sake of your joints and your overall health.

GINGER: GOOD FOR WHAT "ALES" YOUR JOINTS

Ginger is strong medicine against arthritis. It contains potent anti-inflammatory compounds called *gingerols* that have a chemical structure similar to NSAIDs.

■ A study conducted at Miami Medical School involving arthritis patients found that ginger, taken twice daily, reduces pain as effectively as anti-inflammatory drugs.

■ In two other separate clinical studies, doctors found that 75% of arthritis patients and 100% of patients with muscle pain experienced significant relief and reduction in swollen joints after consuming ginger.

■ During another 2 1/2 year clinical trial using powdered ginger on patients with RA and OA, researchers found that approximately 75% of the patients experienced pain relief and decreased swelling, with no reports of adverse effects.

■ Similar studies examining the active ingredient in ginger extract showed that it significantly inhibited the activity of COX-2 and *tumor necrosis factor-alpha* (TNF-a), a nasty inflammatory agent produced by the body. Evidence indicates that TNF plays an important role, not only in inflammatory arthritis, but also in degenerative joint disease.

Look for old-fashioned "ginger beer" in your natural foods market and check the label to make sure it contains real ginger. (Commercial "ginger ale" generally contains no ginger at all, only artificial flavoring.) As little as two to three teaspoons of fresh ginger or ginger powder daily is enough to provide an anti-inflammatory benefit. Brew it as a tea or add the shredded fresh root to recipes. Ginger is also well-known for soothing an upset stomach, just in case your arthritis medication or pain-reliever causes gastrointestinal problems.

JOINT-HEALING JUICE FROM THE BIBLE

The juice of the pomegranate, a fruit mentioned in the Bible, is taking the medical community by storm. In addition to its proven ability to reduce artery plaque and reverse prostate cancer, pomegranate juice contains powerful anti-inflammatory and antioxidant compounds that defend joint cartilage.

When researchers at Case Western Reserve University of Cleveland dripped pomegranate extract on damaged cartilage tissue in the lab, they found it reduced the levels of an enzyme responsible for inflammation. More studies are ongoing, but there are so many marvelous benefits already linked to this wonder-working nectar that there's no reason to wait. And you don't need much – a couple of ounces of unsweetened pomegranate juice per day will do the trick.

Be sure to choose juice with no added sugar. Some brands try to fool you by loudly proclaiming "100% juice" on their label. But this is a dead giveaway that other juices (usually apple) are the main ingredient, with pomegranate having a minor role (sometimes only 10% or less). Real pomegranate juice can be a little strong, which is why we either sweeten it with a little D-ribose [2] or dilute it with soda water to create a sparkling cocktail. Shoot for two to four ounces daily, blending some into your morning smoothie.

---

[2] **D-ribose** (or simply ribose) is a simple, five-carbon sugar found naturally in our bodies. Different from other sugars, it is vital in the production of *adenosine triphosphate* (ATP), which is the energy molecule that powers our hearts, muscles, brains, and every other organ in the body. (ATP is the chemical name for the life force that powers our cells). If a cell has insufficient ribose, it cannot make sufficient ATP. Muscles (including the heart) aren't capable of making ribose very efficiently. Under situations of oxygen deprivation, when chronic exertion and fatigue besiege the heart, congestive heart failure (CHF) can set in and lead to death. Clinical research shows that giving ribose to energy-deficient hearts stimulates energy recovery. I've had a number of patients miraculously recover from CHF by giving them ribose and other heart-energizing supplements (details in my book, *The Sinatra Solution*). Many athletes now take ribose to speed their recovery after endurance exercise.

CHERRY JUICE REDUCES PAIN AND INFLAMMATION

Cherries make a great pie, but a pain-reliever? You bet! Cherries contain powerful natural anti-inflammatory compounds called *anthocyanins* and other flavonoids that work on the same inflammation pathways as aspirin and NSAIDs to reduce pain. Researchers at Michigan State University found that just 10 tart cherries pack the same pain-relieving wallop as one or two aspirin, in addition to their impressive antioxidants.

Cherries also relieve gout, a painful cousin of arthritis. Gout is caused by a buildup of uric acid, which crystallizes in joints and causes pain, stiffness and inflammation. Research at the University of California Davis demonstrated that eating eight ounces of cherries significantly reduced levels of uric acid. Cherries also produce noteworthy decreases in markers of inflammation.

Jim has had great success with cherry juice in treating his arthritis. This summer gave him an abundant cherry harvest, which he munched for weeks. Jim squeezed the rest into juice (about four gallons total), which he sweetened with a little D-ribose and froze in six-ounce bottles. In the evening, Jim removes one for thawing and sips it in the early morning hours while he's writing.

JIM HEALTHY'S JOINT JUICE™

Here's triple health for nagging, painful arthritis. Brew up this combination of green tea with fresh ginger and mix in a splash of pomegranate or cherry juice for a bonanza of anti-inflammatory benefits.

Makes 4 servings

- 4 cups of water in a tea kettle or pot
- 4 green tea bags, or 4 tablespoons of green tea leaves (use a tea ball)
- Fresh ginger, sliced (about the size of your thumb, or more if you like)
- Unsweetened pure pomegranate or cherry juice, to taste.

1. Bring the water to a boil and add the ginger slices. Boil for an additional 30-60 seconds. Remove from the heat, and add the tea bags or tea ball. Let steep for 2 to 3 minutes. No-work "solar brew" alternative: double (or triple) the ginger and tea and place in a one-gallon glass jar or jug. Let it brew in the sun for a few hours.

2. Add pomegranate juice. Sweeten to taste with no-cal stevia[3] or a little honey, but we like to use a half-teaspoon of D-ribose per cup as a mild sweetener because it will support ATP production at the same time. (Increased ATP is the best way to repair weakened or damaged cells.) Sip it hot -- or let it cool in the fridge so you'll always have a refreshing, joint-healing beverage on hand to slake your thirst and keep your joints hydrated.

---

[3] **Stevia** *(Stevia rebaudiana)* is a member of the suflower family and native to South and Central America, where it is commonly known as sweet leaf or sugarleaf. Stevia extract is 300 times sweeter than sugar and has zero calories. Because stevia has a negligible effect on blood glucose, it is used as a natural sweetener for people on carbohydrate-controlled diets, as well as those being treated for obestity and high blood pressure. Widely used as a sweetener in Japan, stevia has been banned in the US as a food ingredient since the early 1990s, although it is legally sold as a supplement. Rebiana is a trade name for a sweetener containing mainly the steviol glycoside *rebaudioside.* Truvia is the brand name of a zero-calorie stevia sweetener marketed by Cargill and developed jointly with the Coca-Cola Company. In December, 2008, the USDA permitted certain stevia-based sweeteners to be used as food additives. When shopping, experiment until you find a product you like. Some have a bitter or licorice-like aftertaste at high concentrations.

(-)

DAY 6: SUBTRACT ONE SODA

HURTER: **Drink one less soda or sugary drink per day than you usually do. This will improve your joint health, decrease your inflammation, help you lose weight and ease your pain.**

SUGAR IS BAD for arthritis in at least four ways – and all four of these negatives involve increased levels of inflammation in your body…

Sugar creates free radicals. In the book Sugar Shock, which I co-authored with Connie Bennett, I describe research done by the eminent endocrinologist Dr. Paresh Dandona at the State University of New York at Buffalo, who demonstrated that drinking sugary beverages increases inflammation and free radical generation immediately after consumption. These free radicals are highly reactive and damage healthy cells and tissues in the body, including joint tissue.

Sugar damages collagen. Sugar molecules attack collagen (one of the main components of cartilage which is responsible for its elasticity and structure) by permanently attaching themselves to its fibers (called cross-linking) and triggering an inflammatory response. This resulting inflammation produces enzymes that break down collagen, making it stiff and inflexible where it was once soft and supple. These "sugar bonds" in collagen generate more free radicals leading to even greater inflammation and deterioration.

Sugar accelerates the aging process. Drinking or eating sugary foods causes a sudden spike in blood glucose which triggers the body's insulin response. Insulin's job is to convert any glucose calories you don't immediately burn as fuel into fat for storage in fat cells. When glucose and insulin levels are chronically elevated (which occurs when you

33

eat or drink lots of sugary foods and drinks), storage cells grow resistant to insulin and the pancreas is forced to pump out more of it. Eventually, the pancreas tires and insulin production wears out, requiring insulin injections. At this point, full-blown diabetes has set in. What does diabetes have to do with arthritis? Plenty…

Elevated levels of sugar and insulin in the bloodstream produce inflammatory waste products called *advanced glycation end products* (AGEs), which accelerate the aging of all tissues in the body. (On the skin, they're seen as "age spots.") In cartilage, AGEs interfere with the normal repair and rebuilding of cartilage because these waste products accumulate. It's like trying to remodel a house without cleaning up the demolition every day. Eventually, the builders won't be able to get into the house at all.

It's no coincidence that people with diabetes (who have much higher levels of AGEs than non-diabetics) also have a greater incidence of OA. But it isn't diabetes that's responsible. Rather, it is chronically high glucose levels caused by overconsumption of sugar.

Sugar makes us fat. In order to store excess glucose calories, insulin must first transform them into fats called *triglycerides* and store them in fat cells, usually around the belly region. And fats cells, particularly in the belly, secrete enzymes which are highly inflammatory.

This is a double-whammy for people with arthritis. Not only does excess sugar add to your body's inflammation, but the extra pounds stress your weight-bearing joints. The famous Framingham Study found a conclusive link between OA and obesity: the more that people weighed, the more likely they were to have or develop OA. Knees and hips normally handle loads equivalent to 2.5 to ten times a person's weight. If you weigh 200 pounds, your joints may be handling as much as one *ton* of pressure as you walk, run or climb stairs! Ten extra pounds feels like 100 to your weight-bearing joints.

Research shows that simply losing weight greatly reduces a person's chances of developing OA, while relieving OA symptoms and discomfort. Does that mean we're going to put you on a diet? *No way.* Besides, diets don't work – and most people rarely stick with them.

But we *will* give you one simple secret that can reduce your weight, slim your body and lower your inflammation levels – and it's just about the easiest thing you can do…

SKIP ONE SODA OR SOFT DRINK PER DAY

Sounds like such a small thing, but it can yield big rewards. These days, sweetened foods and beverages represent 25% of the calories in the typical American diet – with sodas, soft drinks and "juicy drinks" accounting for the lion's share. It's not uncommon for some people to drink three or more of these beverages in a day. And we're not talking about the typical 12-oz. can. Most fountain sodas contain two to three time that amount, which is an avalanche of calories (and potential inflammation). Let's do the math so you can see the impact…

A typical 12-oz. soda contains about 150 calories, so three of these regular-size drinks add up to almost 500 calories. Three modest sodas per day for a week equals roughly 3,500 calories, or the number of calories needed to add one pound of fat to your body. At that rate, a modest soda habit can add *four* extra pounds to a person's weight in one month. No wonder over 65% of US adults are overweight, and more than one in three people are obese. That's over 66 million Americans! Obviously, sodas are not the sole culprit – but they lead the list of sugary foods that are making us fat. And they are also one of the main inflammation-producers.

WE CONSUME OUR WEIGHT IN SUGAR ANNUALLY!

Historical records from 200 years ago show that Americans consumed about 8.4 pounds of sugar per person annually back then – or about 2.2 teaspoons daily. Today, that number has spiked to *one cup*, or 170 pounds per year! And that doesn't include the "hidden sugars" in our food supply.

If that fact didn't make your eyeballs pop, this might: corn sweeteners, mainly high fructose corn syrup (HFCS) add another 83.5 pounds of "sweet inflammation" per person to this intake.

Some of the nation's top obesity researchers at prestigious institutions such as Harvard and Yale have gone on record to say that sodas and other sweetened soft drinks are the leading cause of obesity in today's diet. And a number of studies directly link soft drink consumption to weight gain and obesity. One found that for each additional sweet drink consumed per day, the odds of obesity increased 60%. A Harvard study of 50,000 nurses found that women who drink more sodas regularly have larger increases in their body-mass index (BMI).

The big problem, scientists say, is that calories from sugar-sweetened beverages are not metabolized well by the body. HFCS, the main sweetener now used by the soft drink industry, increases *triglycerides* in the blood because it doesn't trigger an insulin response to get the sugar out of the bloodstream. This raises a person's risk of diabetes, heart disease and other weight-related health problems

The American Journal of Clinical Nutrition reports that another difficulty with HFCS is that it doesn't produce the feeling of satiety (satisfaction) in the brain, so people tend to eat more when a soda accompanies food. HFCS calories have no effect on appetite, making it easier to over-consume.

In animal studies, mice drinking fructose-sweetened water and soft drinks gained 90% more body fat than mice consuming just water because their brains didn't register the HFCS calories. The same phenomenon occurs in humans. Penn State nutritionist Barbara Rolls set up a study in which women were given either water, diet soda, regular soda, orange juice, milk, or no drink before lunch. After eating lunch, the total food intake was 104 calories greater for those given sweetened beverages compared to those given either other beverages or none at all. Clearly, the HFCS soft drinks didn't help women feel any fuller.

HOW SODAS WEAKEN YOUR BONES

Sodas, especially colas, contain *phosphoric acid,* which leaches minerals from bones and leads to osteoporosis. This acid also inhibits your body's ability to absorb the trace mineral *manganese.* Low levels of this mineral significantly weaken the stabilizing ligaments that surround and support joints, making them unstable and subject to an increased risk of subluxation, dislocation, and injury.

If you follow The Arthritis Healing Diet™ (which you'll be introduced to in these 30 days), you'll be receiving sufficient amounts of manganese as long as you aren't blocking its absorption by drinking sodas. Foods richest in manganese include pineapple, spinach, mustard and collard greens, brown rice, and various beans and legumes – all of which help suppress inflammation and contribute to joint healing. For added insurance, make sure your multivitamin contains at least 5 mg of this important mineral.

LOSE ONE SODA – LOSE ONE POUND

"Decreasing soft drink consumption seems to be a promising strategy for preventing and treating obesity," say researchers at the University of Texas Southwestern Medical Center in Dallas. Jim and I heartily agree.

According to our calorie math above, drinking one less soda per day will save you about 1,000 calories per week (the equivalent of a 10-mile walk). That totals 4,000 calories per month—more than enough to lose (or not gain) one pound. In a year's time, that adds up to 12 pounds. And this isn't hypothetical. Studies with teens actually produced these weight reductions.

This isn't brain surgery. Anyone can drink one less soft drink daily. In fact, it's the easiest way we know to begin taking a load off your joints and turn down the inflammation in your body. We're betting that once you see how easy this is—and feel the difference it makes in your arthritis—you'll want to eliminate even more of these inflammation-activating beverages. (Doing that could reduce your weight by one pound per *month* – or 12 pounds per year! – without ever breaking a sweat.)

HIDDEN BENEFITS OF THE ARTHRITIS HEALING DIET™

You bought this book to improve your arthritis, but you're in for an even bigger surprise: you're going to discover a "new you" at the end of this 30-day experiment. You're going to weigh less without dieting. Have more energy without seeing a doctor. Feel calmer, happier and more positively enthusiastic than you have in years. Move with more grace and less pain. Improve your memory and mental function. Sleep better. Pep up your sex life. And that's just for starters.

How is this possible? Easy. In the process of healing your arthritis, you're going to be healing your whole being. That's because inflammation is the bad guy driving most chronic and degenerative diseases. So reducing your levels of inflammation will produce positive consequences in your brain, your arteries, your liver, and your entire body—including your joints.

Another thing: the arthritis healing foods and secrets you'll discover in the days ahead are also great for your overall health.   Step-by-step, you'll be improving many important aspects of your well-being.

Meanwhile, here are some suggestions for arthritis-friendly beverages you can substitute for that one soda or soft drink you'll be forsaking for the health of your joints…

10 ARTHRITIS-FRIENDLY SODA ALTERNATIVES

These 10 suggestions will help you widen your thirst-quenching horizon, reduce your soda habit, and leave your taste buds satisfied.   Since you probably won't find these in any vending machine or convenience store, carry them with you in a small thermos so they stay cool.   Add these to the "Just What the Doctor Ordered" Arthritis Tea you learned about on Day 5. For more free Arthritis Healing Beverages, visit our website at www.myhealingkitchen.com.

1. **Water.** Too boring? Add slices of your favorite fruits and veggies — lemons, oranges, watermelon, cucumber, mint, or limes — to a pitcher of ice-cold water for a refreshing and flavorful drink. Carry your own supply with you wherever you go.

2. **Soda or juice spritzer.** If the idea of going cold turkey is too scary, dilute your favorite soda or juice with ½ to ☐ sparkling water.

3. **Ice ginger or herbal tea.** Sweeten with a little D-ribose, agave syrup, or no-cal stevia.

4. **Chilled green or black tea.** Both are loaded with arthritis-improving nutrients. Sweeten with a little D-ribose or no-cal stevia.

5. **Low-fat milk.** The calcium will help strengthen your bones.

6. **Ice coffee.** But this doesn't mean a 16-ounce Starbucks Caffe Mocha with whipped cream. That packs a whopping 330 calories.

7. **Fruit spritzer.** Mix ¼ unsweetened fruit juice with ¾ sparkling water.

8. **No-cal lemonade**. Sweeten with a little D-ribose or no-cal stevia.

9. **Unsweetened fruit juice**. Pomegranate and cherry are especially good for relieving arthritis pain.

10. **Soy milk.** You can buy it flavored (we both like vanilla) or make your own by blending in your favorite fruit, such as berries, a little banana, or some pineapple.

(+)

DAY 7: TAKE A SUN BATH

HEALER: **Get 10-20 minutes of "sunshine vitamin D" every day on as much of your bare skin as you're comfortable exposing. It's healing for both OA and RA – and it's free!**

YOU'VE BEEN AN ARTHRITIS "TIGER" – and you've learned a lot in just one week. In the past six days you've laid the groundwork for the days and weeks of joint healing ahead.

By now you have a safe, reliable pain-reliever that works well for you. You're taking fish oil to control your inflammation. You're beginning to recognize some of the foods and beverages that are arthritis "pain antagonizers"—and are thinking twice before you reach for them. And you have a number of arthritis-healing beverages to quench your thirst instead of turning to junky, sugary sodas and soft drinks.

Whew! You've been busy. So now on the seventh day, you get to rest. That's right. You're going to improve the condition of your joints and heal your arthritis by lying down and relaxing for ten to 20 minutes … *in the sun*. (And sunscreen isn't allowed!)

HOW THE SUN HEALS ARTHRITIS

You probably know that vitamin D is vital for strong bone strength, but it is also essential for *joint* health…

■ Clinical studies clearly show that vitamin D improves both RA and OA.

■ Furthermore, research shows that people with OA who have a vitamin D deficiency develop greater disability.

■ Other studies indicate that getting adequate amounts of vitamin D preserves muscle strength, improves physical functioning, and retards the deterioration of cartilage.

■ Research has shown that vitamin D reduces inflammation, the sneaky villain behind OA, as well as heart disease, diabetes, and high blood pressure, plus prostate and colon cancers. Research has linked low vitamin D levels to an increased risk of these diseases – and doctors believe a deficiency in this anti-inflammatory nutrient is the reason why.

DON'T BE CAUGHT "D"-FICIENT

Surprise: the majority of Americans are vitamin D deficient. In fact, vitamin D is the leading nutritional deficiency in our nation. Up to 90% of all Americans are deficient in this critical vitamin and scientists estimate that 600,000 cases of cancer in the US could be prevented every year simply by increasing our levels. But the word is not getting out – and most doctors are completely unaware of the problem or the importance of this nutrient.

Vitamin D deficiency has hit epidemic levels and is spreading around the globe. One study revealed that 75% of all men are stricken, while other research indicates that 70% of women 51-70 years old and 90% of women over 70 are affected. In addition to the diseases just mentioned, studies show that vitamin D deficiency significantly increases the risk of dying from all causes.

"WHO, ME?"

How is it that so many of us could be so dangerously deficient in vitamin D? Because we've been told that the sun is harmful. Yet solar rays are the primary source of vitamin D. Your body produces it when the sun's ultraviolet (UV) rays penetrate the skin, with lighter skin producing more of it than darker skin.

Millions of Americans are avoiding sunshine these days because popular health advice says that it causes skin cancer. In addition, they are being told to avoid eating vitamin D rich foods, such as organ meats, such as calves liver, animal fats, dairy foods, and eggs.

BOTH PIECES OF ADVICE ARE DEAD WRONG

Research confirms that vitamin D deficiency increases the risk of death from all causes, *including* skin cancer and melanoma.   In fact, because solar rays are the most significant source of vitamin D for humans – and vitamin D protects against many cancers, including skin cancer – people who get less sun actually have *higher* rates of the skin cancer, melanoma, and other cancers.

Sunscreens, which we are told to slather on ourselves and our children before going outdoors, blocks vitamin D production by 95%. The tragic irony is that people are staying out of the sun to avoid skin cancer and melanoma, but these are two of the main cancers that vitamin D prevents. (Incidentally, studies show that men who expose themselves to sunshine are better protected against prostate cancer.)

DON'T BE A "SOLAR SCARDY CAT"

Besides being turned into "solar scardy cats," we are being steered away from eating foods that are rich in vitamin D. Check the Top Ten list below and you'll see that consumption of the top food sources – organ meats, animal fats, dairy foods, and eggs – is being discouraged by doctors and mainstream health advice. These are the same "experts" who are telling us to stay out of the sun.

The Top 10 Vitamin D Foods:

1. Liver and other organ meats
2. Wild salmon (not farm-raised)
3. Shrimp
4. Cod
5. Anchovies
6. Fish oil
7. Eggs
8. Milk (fortified)
9. Red, yellow, and orange fruits and vegetables
10. Dark-green, leafy vegetables

SHOULD YOU TAKE A SUPPLEMENT?

Getting 100% of your vitamin D requirements from food sources is difficult because foods are a poor source. Most people will need to take supplements when sunbathing isn't possible (in winter, for instance). In this case, a vitamin D supplement is you best insurance. Here are some important shopping tips…

■ If you opt for a supplement, purchase only a high-quality brand of vitamin D3 (*cholecalciferol*). This is the same form of vitamin D that our skin produces from sunlight. Good old cod liver oil works just as well.

■ By all means avoid vitamin D2 (*ergocalciferol*) because it is inferior and potentially harmful. The human body was never meant to receive vitamin D in this form because it isn't present in breast milk.

■ And speaking of babies, here's an astounding fact underscoring the importance of vitamin D: studies show that infants who get the highest levels of vitamin D (usually through sun exposure) develop 80% less Type 2 diabetes as adults.

■ You should take a minimum of 1,000-2,000 IU of vitamin D3 on days when you cannot expose your body to sunshine. African-Americans, who have higher cancer rates and lower blood levels of vitamin D, should double this dose. (The skin of African Americans does not seem to convert UV rays into vitamin D very well either, which causes a chronic deficiency, particularly among those living in the West. This helps explain why African-Americans generally display a higher incidence of many cancers and in more aggressive forms.)

■ Attention, seniors: your body's ability to produce vitamin D declines with age. A 70-year-old's skin makes about a quarter of the vitamin D that it manufactured from the sun's rays when they were in their 20's. So seniors should take 2,000-3,000 daily, too.

■ Don't worry about doctors who warn of "vitamin D toxicity" – they are behind the research curve. The most recent studies confirm that doses as high as 10,000 IU a day are unlikely to be harmful, though you probably would never want to take this much.

The danger of vitamin D toxicity begins around 20,000 IU per day, and then only if taken for prolonged periods.

THE MOST IMPORTANT NUTRIENT FOR HEALTH AND HEALING?

It's difficult to rank nutrients by their importance because so many are essential and often work in combination. But if I had to place one healing nutrient at the top of my list, it would be vitamin D. Unique from other vitamins, D affects the entire body. Receptors that respond to it occur in every human cell, from your brain to your bones. Though classified as a vitamin, it acts more like a hormone in the body. Scientists are only beginning to understand how important vitamin D is for the optimal health and healing of a wide range of conditions.

BONE UP ON SUNSHINE VITAMIN D

Lying in the sun feels good because it *is* good for you. Solar rays nurture all life, and we humans are no exception. Scientists have yet to identify the many ways that sunshine helps heal us, but when I'm ill, I like to recuperate in the sun's warmth and fresh air. Sun exposure was a popular therapy for tuberculosis before the advent of TB vaccination. It is now believed that patients got well because of increased blood levels of healing vitamin D.

Until we learn more about the sun's effect of health and healing, beyond the production of vitamin D – we should do as our ancestors did and expose our skin to the sun instead of hiding from it.

Amazing fact: most people believe that staying out of the sun lowers their risk of skin cancer -- but just the opposite is true. Studies show that lily-whites have *higher* rates of skin cancer and melanoma than people who are moderately-tanned, as long as they do not experience sunburn. The extra vitamin D makes the difference.

...AND IT'S FREE!

You won't need to spend a penny either, because the best source of vitamin D is sunshine. The current solar hysteria and wrinkle-phobia sweeping the US is making sunscreen manufacturers and dermatologists wealthier, but it's also creating a wave of vitamin D deficiency that is making OA a bigger problem for people who have it. If you can, bathe in the sun for up to 20 minutes every day. It's some of the best medicine you can take – and it's absolutely free.

Take care not to burn because sunburn generates free radicals and is linked to skin cancer. (Set an alarm or ask your partner to arouse you just in case you should fall asleep.) Don't wear sunscreen unless you're going to be in the sun for longer periods. When winter approaches and it's too cold to go outside, use a supplement.

(–)

DAY 8: CEASE THE CEREALS

HURTER: **Cut back on (or eliminate) processed breakfast cereals, toast, muffins, Pop-Tarts, donuts, pastries and any other popular cereal-based breakfast foods you may be eating, because they tend to inflame your joints.**

IF YOU HAVE ARTHRITIS, either OA or RA, it's important to reduce your intake of refined carbohydrate foods, particularly breakfast cereals, breads, muffins, donuts, and pastries. These are definitely *not* part of The Arthritis Healing Diet™. Quite the opposite – they are highly inflammatory and can make your joints hurt worse. Here's why…

REFINED CARBS TRIGGER THE INFLAMMATION RESPONSE

Your body responds to refined carbohydrates the same as if you'd eaten sugar. Both generate spikes in glucose and insulin, which are highly inflammatory. Refined carbs also prompt your body to release *cytokines*, proteins that regulate the body's inflammation response. Inflammation makes arthritis worse, period. It not only worsens joint soreness and stiffness, but raises the risk of heart attack, diabetes, Alzheimer's, cancer, and artery disease. And here are some other reasons refined carbs are bad for your joints…

Too many omega-6s. Most processed foods also contain refined vegetable oils, such as soy, corn, cottonseed, or canola, which are rich in pro-inflammatory omega-6 fatty acids. (You learned about this danger on Day 4.) So, with processed foods – especially baked goods – you're getting a double-whammy.

To keep inflammation to a minimum, your diet should maintain a ratio of omega-6s to omega-3s around 1:1 or 2:1. Incredibly, the typical American diet is about 20:1. That's a big reason we are experiencing so many inflammation-driven diseases today. Consider this: the incidence of arthritis in the US has risen dramatically since the early 1900s, when our diet began to change from natural whole foods to the processed type which could be preserved in boxes and bags on grocer's shelves.

Wheat allergy. Many people with OA and RA have secret allergies to – and intolerance of – wheat products. This can cause inflammatory flare-ups and painful misery. You'll read more about this in the days ahead – and discover a simple way to tell if this is causing problems for you … plus how to stop it. (If you suspect you have a wheat allergy, jump ahead to Day 28 to read what you can do about it).

Fewer inflammation-fighting foods. At the same time, if you're mostly consuming processed foods, it usually means you're eating fewer of the foods shown to have anti-inflammatory effects. Try to remember this the next time you reach for boxed breakfast cereals, baked goods, coffee cakes, or a donut. It's like begging for more pain in your joints.

THE EASY SOLUTION

To control inflammation and joint pain, build your breakfast around whole foods and fresh produce, such as whole grains, coarse, steel-cut oatmeal, fresh fruits, "lean-and-clean" protein, free-range chicken eggs, yogurt, and other healthful dairy foods, plus nuts, seeds, and soy foods. These should comprise the majority of your meal. It's easier to add more good foods to your diet than to fight your cravings for the bad ones.

Rule of thumb: Eat foods as close to their natural state as possible. Choose oatmeal instead of an oat bran muffin. Here's why! The muffin is made of refined flour, lots of vegetable oil and a big dollop of sugar or other sweeteners. On the other hand, oatmeal is one of nature's perfect healing foods. It's hearty, satisfying, loaded with healing nutrients, and chockfull of fiber. That high fiber content slows the release of glucose in your bloodstream, requiring less insulin, and providing a steady flow of glucose to fuel your body and brain all morning. Top it off with some fresh berries, yogurt, and ground flaxseed, and you'll have a perfect anti-arthritis breakfast to keep your joints calm and pain-free. If you're still unsure what *not* to eat, try to consume fewer of the foods on this list:

The Top 10 Worst Refined Carbs in the US Diet:

1. Bread (non-whole grain)
2. Soft drinks and all sugary beverages, including sports drinks
3. Cakes, cookies and doughnuts
4. Any food with sugar or high fructose corn syrup
5. Jams and jellies
6. Boxed breakfast cereals
7. White rice, white-flour pasta
8. Fruit juice "drinks"
9. Frozen desserts
10. Chips and crackers

Go easy on (or completely avoid) foods that come from a box or that have unrecognizable ingredients on the label. The more you limit your consumption of these commercial breakfast "foods," the better your joints will feel. And that means less pain and more flexibility.

THEY ALSO HELP YOU LOSE WEIGHT

Whole foods fill you up faster because they're nutrient-dense, meaning they pack a lot of nutritional punch and fiber without many calories. This will keep your weight in check and minimize the stress on your weight-bearing knees and hips. According to the National Health and Nutrition Examination Survey, women who are obese have four times the risk of OA of the knee than women who weigh less. And for men, the risk is nearly five times greater. Every extra pound can *quadruple* the load on your joints – and that can hurt. On the bright side, every pound you lose removes four pounds of pressure from your hips and knees.

Losing weight also lowers the level of inflammatory chemicals in your bloodstream, which also eases pain. That's because fat cells, especially those around your belly, secrete pro-inflammatory hormones that raise your blood levels of C-reactive protein (CRP) and makes your joints stiff and sore.

You'll discover other suggestions for inflammation-taming breakfast foods in the days ahead. But for now, feast on fruits and cease the cereals. You'll look and feel a whole lot better.

(+)

DAY 9: HAVE A "BERRY" GOOD BREAKFAST

HEALER: **Here's a breakfast that will fill you up and quiet your hunger until lunch – while calming and soothing your joints as if you munched a bunch of ibuprofen.**

SOME FOODS ARE REAL MEDICINE – and more than 9,000 scientific studies prove it. Scientists are becoming awed by the healing compounds in nature's astonishing "food pharmacy." They've identified natural compounds in certain foods which act like tranquilizers, laxatives, beta-blockers, blood thinners, antidepressants, cholesterol reducers, cancer fighters, vasodilators, insulin regulators, expectorants, antibiotics, digestive aids, and – lucky for those of us who have arthritis – powerful anti-inflammatory agents and analgesic pain-relievers.

In the next 21 days, you're going to discover the most potent of these anti-arthritis foods and how to incorporate them into your Arthritis Healing Diet™ to block the inflammation cycle, increase your comfort, halt the deterioration of the joints, and actually help them heal. Here's the first step...

THE ANTI-ARTHRITIS BREAKFAST OF CHAMPIONS

How many times have you heard breakfast referred to as "the most important meal of the day?" Well, it's true – especially so for people with arthritis. You see, depending on what you choose to eat, breakfast can either set you up for a day of sore, stiff, achy joints – or one filled with graceful, easy movement, and comfort.

Some foods, as you've begun to learn, trigger inflammation throughout the body especially in arthritic joints. But other foods have just the opposite effect: they block inflammation by flooding your bloodstream with natural anti-inflammatory compounds that work just like pain-blocking prescription medications, but without any of their side effects.

And topping the list are cherries and berries, which is why I start my day with a heaping bowl of them topped with yogurt and ground flaxseed. For my money, this is the world's best anti-arthritis breakfast. Let me explain...

THE WORLD'S GREATEST PAIN-RELIEVING FRUITS

Cherries and berries aren't just sweet treats; they're also loaded with natural pain-relievers and joint-healing substances. For one thing, they are Nature's richest sources of *anthocyanins*, a group of antioxidants (called *flavonoids*) that possesses exceptional anti-inflammatory properties. That's why blueberries, blackberries, raspberries, strawberries, and cherries head my list of anti-arthritis fruits.

Having pain-free joints is as easy as eating a half cup of mixed berries and cherries daily to maintain high levels of joint-protective antioxidants in your bloodstream. Tart cherries, for example, are ten times more active than aspirin for joint pain. Scientists at Michigan State University found that just 20 tart cherries contain 25 mg of anthocyanins, enough to block the COX-2 enzyme that makes arthritic joints hurt, while reducing inflammation the same way that NSAID drugs do.

Think of red and blue berries are Nature's "pain pills." These two color pigments are telltale signs of the highest anthocyanin content, and are able to deliver a knockout punch to those devilish free radical molecules that initiate and aggravate arthritis pain and joint destruction. Anthocyanins also support the production of healthy collagen, which is the infrastructure of all connective tissue, especially in your joints.

CLINICAL STUDIES PROVE IT

At Baylor University, scientists conducted a study to test the effect of cherry extract on people with arthritis. They found that five out of six participants experienced "significant relief" from it. What's more, the cherry extract caused no side effects. After a mere three months, one participant claimed her pain had completely disappeared. But once she stopped the cherry extract, her pain returned, which is why she's now drinking 100% unsweetened cherry juice and enjoying fresh cherries every chance she gets.

Research conducted at the Harvard University School of Public Health discovered that strawberries also drive down levels of *C-reactive protein* (CRP), a blood marker for inflammation that can go sky-high in people with arthritis. The Harvard researchers found that women eating 16 or more fresh or frozen strawberries per week lowered CRP levels by 14%.

OTHER BERRIES THAT RELIEVE ARTHRITIS PAIN

■ Cranberries are incredibly rich in another antioxidant flavonoid called *quercetin*, which also produces strong anti-inflammatory effects in arthritic joints. And the flavonoid content of the humble strawberry is equally remarkable. Studies show that it blocks the pain and inflammation caused by the nasty COX-2 enzyme just as well as high-priced arthritis drugs such as Celebrex. Like these drugs, flavonoids block the pain and inflammation of COX-2 without inhibiting the non-inflammatory COX-l. And strawberries won't produce side effects linked to these popular drugs, such as heart muscle damage and increased risk of heart attack

■ The tiny blueberry is a mighty arthritis-healing force to be reckoned with. It's packed with more antioxidant power than any other vegetable or fruit, according to Tufts University researchers. Wild blueberries are even *more* spectacular, containing at least five different types of anthocyanins. Berries and cherries also provide exceptional cell protection against free radical molecules that damage DNA, cell membranes and joint tissue.

■ Another way berries protect your joints is through their vitamin C content. Research published in the *Annals of the Rheumatic Diseases* show that foods high in vitamin C protect against a specific type of rheumatoid arthritis (RA) called *inflammatory polyarthritis*, a condition in which two or more joints are affected. (Cherries and berries, by the way, are loaded with C.) According to a study of 20,000 people, researchers found that those who didn't eat very many vitamin C-rich foods had 300% more OA and RA than those who ate the most.

HOW TO FIND THE BEST BERRIES

So where can you find these fruits at their best? Michigan's summer tart cherry crop is legendary – and available through the mail. More convenient still, you can check your local farmer's market or farms in your area for fresh berries and cherries. Buy locally-grown berries in bulk during the season and freeze them for the off-season. For your health's sake, insist on fruit that's been grown without pesticides – and support farmers who don't use harmful chemicals. Dried berries and cherries are another good choice, but read labels to ensure they have no added sugar, oils or chemical preservatives.

Berry juice thwarts joint pain, too. Just be sure it's made from organic berries and contains no added sweeteners. Make yourself a refreshing, joint-soothing spritzer by mixing one-part 100% cherry, blueberry, pomegranate, or other berry juice with two-parts sparkling water or seltzer. Go easy on drinking the juice straight because it contains a lot of calories. Eating whole berries is best because they have fewer calories, more fiber, and superior healing properties.

RECIPE FOR A PAIN-FREE DAY

Here's my prescription for an ideal way to start your joint-comfortable day: cover a bowl of fresh mixed berries with "live-culture" low-fat yogurt (vanilla-flavored soy yogurt works well, too) and top with cinnamon and a generous sprinkle of ground flaxseed. Why the yogurt and flaxseed? Because they also are excellent arthritis-fighting foods. (You'll read how and why in the days ahead. Until then, you'll have to trust me on this.)

For a variation, spoon fresh or frozen berries onto oatmeal with cinnamon and a dollop of yogurt. During the off-season, keep frozen cherries and berries on your grocery list and in your freezer. The thawed fruit may not have the flavor-burst of fresh fruit, but it carries the same outstanding joint-healing power. Your arthritis and your taste buds will thank you.

So will your waistline, because berries are an ideal weight-loss food. Reason? They're loaded with fiber, so they keep your stomach full and your bloodstream supplied with a steady stream of glucose for several hours. After a breakfast like this, I usually don't feel any hunger pangs until mid-afternoon. (For a list of my Top 10 "In-A-Hurry" Arthritis-Fighting Breakfasts, plus many more free recipes, go to www.myhealingkitchen.com).

Arthritis "Power Smoothie"
Serves: 1
Prep. Time: 10 minutes

This "in a hurry" breakfast smoothie will keep your joints comfortable all morning. It's packed with four Arthritis Healing Superfoods that are proven to block painful inflammation and protect your joints. In addition, it contains hunger-quashing protein powder and a boatload of fiber to keep your appetite in check with a minimum of calories (so it's great for weight-loss). Your smoothie whips up in minutes and is easily transported in a thermos bottle, so you can sip it during your commute or later in the morning.

INGREDIENTS:

2 cups strawberries, blueberries, blackberries, and raspberries (any combination; fresh or frozen)
1 cup "live cultures" yogurt (low-fat dairy or soy)
2 tablespoons whey protein powder or spirulina powder
1 cup soy milk or unsweetened cherry or pomegranate juice
1-2 tablespoons of ground flaxseed
A few ice cubes (omit if you use frozen berries)

INSTRUCTIONS:

Place all ingredients in blender and blend until smooth. Drink immediately or transfer to a thermos bottle for easy transport. Even easier: Make a bigger batch and freeze in ice cube trays. Transfer frozen "smoothie cubes" to zip-lock bag and store in the freezer. When needed, pop a few cubes into the blender add juice or soy milk and you're good to go!

> **NUTRITION FACTS:** *Calories 449.5, Total Fat 14.3g, Sat. Fat 3.1g, Cholesterol 14.7mg, Sodium 348.2mg, Fiber 14.6g, Sugars 21.3g, Protein 32.1g*

(–)

DAY 10: PASS ON THE PUFAS

HURTER: **Some fats and oils are healing for your joints, while others have the opposite effect. Most people, including those with arthritis, are in the dark about which oils and fats they should be consuming. So let's shed some light on the subject...**

ON DAYS 4 AND 8, you learned about the inflammation-triggering consequences (ouch!) of eating too many omega-6 foods. Today I'm going to introduce you to one of the biggest sources of omega-6s in our modern diet: vegetable-based, polyunsaturated oils (PUFAs), including corn, soybean, cottonseed, safflower, sunflower, and canola. Corn and soybean oil contain 50% omega-6 and almost no omega-3. Canola oil, which is often touted as "the healthy alternative," has 20% omega-6 and 10% omega-3. This may sound like the right balance, but canola oil is unhealthful because, like all PUFAs, it easily oxidizes in the bloodstream and encourages free radical damage, which is directly linked to inflammation and joint damage.

THE BIG FAT LIE

No doubt you've heard how "bad" animal fats and foods are for you, why vegetable oils are so "healthful," and how if you lower your saturated fat and replace it with polyunsaturated oils, you'll be much healthier. Doctors and nutritionists have repeated this standard advice so often it has become like a mantra. But these recommendations are not only wrong, they're harmful. Here's the story...

Beginning in the 1950s health officials began advising us to cut back on or entirely give up foods containing saturated fats (red meat, dairy foods—especially butter—and eggs). In their place we're told to replace them with a host of synthetic and processed foods created in the laboratory from vegetable oils, sugars, and chemicals. Billions of dollars have gone into their development, marketing and promotion as "health foods." Yet they are anything but.

Nutritionists analyzing USDA data found that the most dramatic change in the modern American diet has been a huge increase in the consumption of liquid vegetable oils, from slightly less than 2 grams per person per day in 1909 to over 30 grams in 1993—a 15-fold increase. During this same period Americans also began consuming newly developed processed food products made with vegetable oils, including oleomargarine, which was touted as a low-cost "more healthful" substitute for butter.

The advice about the "healthfulness" of the unsaturated vegetable oils and butter-replacement products was completely unsupported by scientific evidence. Instead, it was a clever marketing scheme by the food industry to bolster the sales of an entirely new category of highly-profitable products with the full support of the medical community.

Just as there are good and bad carbohydrates, certain oils are highly inflammatory, while others are extraordinarily healthful and anti-inflammatory. Numerous population studies show that PUFAs found in vegetable oils are *worse* for our health than saturated fats. Let's examine this a bit more closely…

THE NATURE OF FATS

The standard advice regarding fats dates back to the 1950s, when we first were told to avoid such saturated fats as butter, animal products, and coconut oil, mainly because they were thought to raise cholesterol and cause heart disease. We were also told to substitute the so-called "heart healthy" polyunsaturated fats, such as corn and soybean oils, to reduce our cholesterol. But little was said about monounsaturated fats such as olive oil, because they were thought to have a neutral effect. This information is far from accurate.

Instead of being the dietary pariah it is made out to be, saturated fat is actually a healthy food source that provides valuable fat-soluble vitamins and nutrients that are essential to the body. Polyunsaturated fats, the ones that were supposed to save us from heart disease and cancer, have been a major influence in today's epidemic rates of both conditions. And monounsaturated fats, because of the beneficial role they play in insulin management, are anything but "neutral." In fact, they represent one of the most healthful and healing fats you can eat. Understanding the chemistry of fats will help you see why the current "politically correct" health advice regarding oils is wrong and dangerous. Here is a primer on fats that can help you differentiate the good fats from the bad…

Saturated fat. A fatty acid is "saturated" when all its available carbon bonds are occupied by hydrogen atoms, which makes it highly stable. This stability means it is unlikely to oxidize or trigger inflammation. This molecular composition makes them solid or semi-solid at room temperature. Your body manufactures saturated fats from carbohydrates and they are also present in animal fats and tropical oils, such as coconut and palm.

For nearly five decades, the medical establishment has regarded saturated fats as one of the greatest risks for heart disease. But this claim is not supported by research. In fact, a three-year study of post-menopausal women published in the *American Journal of Clinical Nutrition* showed that saturated fats actually *protected* their arteries and slowed the accumulation of plaque. At the start of the study, researchers took X-rays of the women's heart arteries. The women kept comprehensive records of the foods they ate and how much, including what kinds of oils they used for frying and baking. At the end of the three-year period, researchers took a second set of images and found that women who had regularly eaten the highest amounts of saturated fats had the least additional plaque buildup in their arteries. The saturated fat group also had a healthier balance of good and bad cholesterols. "Whatever is the cause of heart disease," says the eminent UK biochemist Professor Michael Gurr in his classic text, Lipid Biochemistry, "it is not primarily the consumption of saturated fats."

And yet we are constantly scolded (still!) like naughty children and made to feel guilty for desiring some of tastiest, most healthful foods on earth such as artisan cheeses, omelets, and juicy steaks (although people with arthritis should go a bit easy on these foods—and I'll explain why another day).

Not only do these foods excite and satisfy our senses (unlike laboratory-engineered processed foods), but they also serve important biological functions. Both saturated fats and cholesterol provide cell membranes with stiffness and stability. When an excess of polyunsaturated fats are present in the diet, they replace saturated fats in cell membranes, making the cell walls weak and flabby. When the body recognizes this, cholesterol from the blood is drawn into the cell walls to restore their structural integrity. This is why we see a reduction in serum cholesterol levels when saturated fats are replaced by polyunsaturated oils in the diet. But this effect is only temporary.

Monounsaturated fat. The fats in this category lack two hydrogen atoms and tend to be liquid at room temperature, though they solidify when refrigerated. Like saturated fats, they are relatively stable and tend not to oxidize easily. The most common food source of monounsaturated fatty acid is *oleic acid*, founded in the oils of olives, almonds, avocados, pecans, cashews, peanuts, and other nuts. Monounsaturated fat is the main fat in the Mediterranean Diet, which has been shown in virtually every research study to be associated with lower levels of heart disease and cancer, not to mention longer life spans. But in the 1950s, the medical community was certain that saturated fats increased total cholesterol, while polyunsaturated fats decreased it. The health benefits of monounsaturated fats were unrecognized until the late 1970s, when researchers discovered that monounsaturated fats were highly heart-protective because they raise HDL and lower LDL.

Polyunsaturated fats. This is the most unstable form of fatty acid because it lacks four or more hydrogen atoms, making it highly susceptible to oxidation and spoilage. The two most common food sources of PUFAs found in our foods are *omega-6 linoleic acid* and *omega-3 linolenic acid*. Since our bodies cannot manufacture them, they are referred to as "essential" fatty acids (EFAs) and must be obtained from our diet. The greater the degree of unsaturation in a fatty acid (i.e., the more double bonds it contains), the more vulnerable it is to lipid *peroxidation*, commonly known as rancidity.

Because EFAs are highly reactive, and none more so than the omega-3s, they must be stored and treated with care. That's why polyunsaturated oils, including those made from soy, corn, safflower, cottonseed, and canola should be avoided entirely—especially for cooking. Given what we know today, it is scandalous that these oils continue to dominate our food supply and are still widely present in baked goods, processed foods, and salad dressings.

The ease with which these oils become rancid in the body is the main reason they cause so many health problems. Their oxidation creates a barrage of free radical molecules that attack cell membranes, joints, artery linings, and DNA/RNA strands. This leads to artery disease, cancers, Alzheimer's, cataracts, and arthritis, plus wrinkles and premature aging. This proliferation of free radicals also robs the body of its protective antioxidant supplies, which exacerbates these health problems and weakens the immune system.

Standard health advice recommends that you substitute polyunsaturated oils for the saturated fats in your diet and that they comprise approximately 30% of your calories. But highly-reliable scientific research confirms that this is bad advice. Studies show that PUFAs should be no greater than *four percent* of your total calories and should come directly from food sources such as grains, nuts, green vegetables, and fish, but *not* from commercial vegetable oils.

CUT BACK ON OMEGA-6S

Another reason why PUFA oils are troublesome is because they contain too much omega-6 linoleic acid and too little omega-3. As you've learned, excess omega-6 in the diet has been found to interfere with the production of prostaglandins, hormone-like substances that help reduce inflammation. Research shows that this disruption can result in increased inflammation, high blood pressure, cancer, weight gain, and immune system dysfunction.

Much of this has to do with how our bodies evolved. For millions of years, our ancestors ate diets of roughly a one-to-one ratio of omega-6s to omega-3s, so that's what our bodies are designed to handle. Today, the ratio has shifted dramatically, with the average American consuming at least 15-20 parts omega-6s to one part omega-3s.

As you've already discovered, omega-3 fatty acids have powerful anti-inflammatory effects in the body and their absence in our diet is a significant reason for the current epidemic proportions of inflammatory-based diseases such as arthritis, cardiovascular disease, diabetes, asthma, Alzheimer's, and many cancers.

Eating foods that have too many omega-6s and too few omega-3s poses a health problem because both fats fight for the same enzymes to activate their inflammatory and anti-inflammatory effects in the body. When you eat a food that contains more omega-6s and fewer omega-3s, the omega-6s use up the available enzymes in order to produce inflammatory compounds, which prevent the manufacture of anti-inflammatory prostaglandins, thromboxanes, and leukotrienes. The result is a tendency toward inflammation throughout the body.

Unfortunately, the American diet is awash in inflammation-causing omega-6s, mainly in the form of these PUFA vegetable oils. In addition, refined vegetable oils such as soybean oil are widely used in processed foods, including crackers, cookies, and other snack foods, as well as fast foods. Americans eat so many of these omega-6 "foods" that experts estimate a staggering 20% of their calories come from high omega-6 soybean oil alone.

PASS ON THE REFINED VEGETABLE OILS— AND FOODS THAT CONTAIN THEM

You can improve your balance of omega-6s and omega-3s by reducing your consumption of polyunsaturated oils and processed foods that contain them. You'll also want to up your intake of foods rich in omega-3s, such as fish and ground flaxseed. Another way is to upgrade the quality of the meat you're eating, either by consuming more wild game or choosing beef and poultry that has spent its entire life grazing in pastures. According to a study done at Iowa State University, truly free-range cattle have an omega-3 content on a level that compares with some fish.

So how can you cut back on omega-6s to improve your ration of 6s to 3s? The fastest and easiest way is to stop eating all fast foods and processed foods, and to cease using PUFA vegetable oils when you prepare food. (That includes commercial salad dressings.)

Safflower, corn, sunflower, soybean, and cottonseed oils each contain over 50% omega-6 and, except for soybean oil, only minimal amounts of omega-3. Use of these oils should be strictly limited. They should never be consumed raw or after they've been heated, as in cooking, frying, or baking. High-oleic safflower and sunflower oils, which are produced from hybrid plants, have a composition similar to olive oil, namely, high amounts of oleic acid and only small amounts of polyunsaturated fatty acids and, thus, are more stable than traditional varieties. However, it is nearly impossible to find truly cold-pressed versions of these oils.

THE CANOLA OIL HOAX

Canola oil, marketed as the "healthy alternative," is no better than the rest—and may actually be worse. Processed from a hybrid strain of rapeseed, hydrogenated shortening made from canola oil can contain as much as 50% TRANS-fat. It goes rancid easily and baked goods that contain it quickly become moldy. During the deodorizing process, the omega-3 fatty acids of processed canola oil are transformed into TRANS-fats, similar to those in margarine and possibly more dangerous. A recent study indicates that canola oil creates a vitamin E deficiency in the body, which encourages free radical proliferation.

Modern refining methods make matters worse. In pre-industrial times, oil was extracted from fruits, nuts, and seeds by slow-moving stone presses, a process referred to as "cold pressing" that preserves their health-promoting saturated linolenic acid, as well as their natural vitamin E content. Modern oil processing is extremely harsh by comparison and destroys much of the oil's inherent nutritional quality. After high-pressure crushing, the oil is heated to 230 degrees and exposed to oxygen and light, which creates dangerous free radicals. In order to extract the last 10% of oil from the crushed seeds, the pulp is then treated with a toxic solvent that is boiled off, although a detectable portion remains. Antioxidants originally present in the seeds, such as vitamin E, are also destroyed and replaced by the preservatives BHT and BHA, both of which have been implicated in causing cancer and brain damage. Don't fall for the hype that canola oil is the "healthy" alternative. It isn't by a long shot.

"SO WHAT OILS SHOULD I USE?"

There are safe, modern techniques that extract monounsaturated oil and its delicate antioxidants under low temperatures. Look for labels that say "expeller-pressed" or "unrefined." These will remain fresh for many years in the refrigerator or if packaged. in opaque containers or dark bottles. Here are some suggestions ...

Flaxseed oil.   One of nature's richest sources of omega-3s, flaxseed oil provides a remedy for today's widespread omega-6/omega-3 imbalance. But because it is so rich in omega-3s, it spoils easily, although new techniques for extraction and bottling have minimized the problem. In Scandinavian countries, flaxseed oil is a valued health remedy. Use it sparingly in salad dressings, never cook with it, and always keep it refrigerated and protected from light.

Peanut oil. Relatively stable at high heat, peanut oil is appropriate for higher heat stir-frying. One caution however: due to its high percentage of omega-6s, use of peanut oil should be limited.

Sesame oil. Similar in composition to peanut oil, it can be used for frying because its unique antioxidants are not destroyed by heat. As with peanut oil, it shouldn't be used frequently because of its high omega-6 content.

Coconut oil.   Tropical oils have fallen victim to the misinformed hysteria surrounding saturated fat. This is unfortunate because their molecular structure allows them to withstand high heat, making them ideal for cooking and baking. Their "bad reputation" is the result of intense lobbying by the vegetable oil industry, which sought to replace coconut oil when it was widely used in cookies, crackers, and pastries.

Conventional health advice claims that consumption of saturated fats can increase the risk of CHD, but a 2004 study published in the journal *Clinical Biochemistry* found that virgin coconut oil actually *reduced* LDL cholesterol, while raising beneficial HDL levels. Other convincing research shows that saturated tropical oils do not contribute to heart disease. Studies done in the 1960s on populations in the Pacific Islands and Asia whose diets are high in coconut oil revealed low levels of CHD, cancers, and other degenerative diseases. My friend and fellow nutritionist Jonny Bowden describes a long-term multidisciplinary study, which examined people living on the coconut-eating islands of Tokelau and Pukapuka in the South Pacific. Although up to 60% of the population's calories came from the saturated fat of coconuts, the Islanders were lean, healthy, and virtually free of atherosclerosis, heart disease, colon cancer, and digestive problems.

The saturated fat in coconut is composed of *medium-chain triglycerides* (MCTs) and is much easier to metabolize than long-chain saturated fats because the body is more likely to use them for energy instead of fat storage. The *Physicians' Desk Reference* describes how MCTs are helpful against some cancers and exhibit positive effects on the immune system. One reason is that coconut oil is extremely rich in *lauric acid*, a natural antiviral and antibacterial compound that also makes mother's milk so protective.

Coconut oil also helps keeps tropical populations relatively free from the disease-causing bacteria and fungi so prevalent in their food supply. As more Third World nations in the tropics have switched to polyunsaturated vegetable oils, the incidence of intestinal disorders and immune deficiency diseases has increased dramatically. On a recent trip to Mexico, I learned that small children harboring parasites are fed coconut water first thing in the morning as an effective remedy.

Coconut oil is also rich in *myristic acid*, an important fatty acid used by your body's immune system to fight tumors through a process called *myristoylation*. Most Westerners are deficient in myristic acid because we are told to avoid coconut oil and its other main dietary source, dairy products.

Palm oil. Along with palm kernel oil, these saturated vegetable fats also contain high levels of lauric acid. Like coconut oil, both are extremely stable and can be kept at room temperature for many months without becoming rancid. Unfortunately, the price of these oils has risen dramatically because of their industrial use. It is a tragedy that many Asian people are being forced to use cheaper polyunsaturated vegetable oils instead.

WHEN SHOPPING FOR OILS

Your choice of fats and oils is one of the most important factors influencing your health. Don't be afraid of saturated fats despite the widespread propaganda suggesting the opposite. The research is very clear on this. The oils to avoid are the PUFAs, such as those made from safflower, corn, sunflower, soybean, cottonseed, and canola because they are high in omega-6s, are highly inflammatory, and oxidize rapidly in the body to create free radicals, which deplete the body of its antioxidants and damage cells, tissues, and organs. Shun any processed foods containing them or any fat that has been "hydrogenated," which is another word for TRANS-fat. Use extra virgin olive oil or small amounts of unrefined flaxseed oil or walnut oil for salad dressings.

Never heat any oil to the point at which it smokes, and avoid inhaling the smoke of any fat because it is toxic and carcinogenic. Any oil is ruined at its smoke point and is no longer good for you. Carefully discard it and start over. That's why I prefer small amounts of coconut or sesame oils for stir-frying because both have a high smoking point and stay molecularly stable during high heat. When baking, stick with coconut oil or animal fats such as butter or lard. (Yes, butter and lard! Contrary to what you've heard, research confirms they are much safer and healthier than polyunsaturated vegetable oils.)

Any oil that has gone rancid is *toxic*. Ingesting it is like pouring free radical molecules into your body. Rancid oil has an unpleasant odor similar to varnish or oil paint. Discard it immediately. To prevent oxidation, buy high-quality oils in small containers and protect them from heat and light.

(+)

DAY 11: GO FISHING FOR HEALTHIER JOINTS

HEALER: **Certain varieties of fish top the list of the most arthritis-healing foods on earth. That's why I recommend you build your anti-arthritis diet around them. Here's the story...**

IF YOU NEED RELIEF from your sore, inflamed arthritic joints, look no further than the fish counter in your local supermarket. Certain varieties of fish possess natural compounds that halt inflammation, relieve pain, and actually encourage your joints to produce new cartilage on par with the top drugs.

HOW OMEGA-3 FISH RELIEVES ARTHRITIS PAIN

Inflammation is responsible for that sore, aching sensation in your knees, hips, shoulders, hands, and spine. Cartilage, you see, has no nerve endings, so you can have raw bone grinding on bone and not feel any pain. What *does* make you hurt, however, is the inflammation that results as your immune system steps in to provide lubrication to ease the friction. These inflammatory fluids contain harsh enzymes called *interleukins* which irritate nerve endings on the inside lining of the synovial sac that surrounds joints. This is what causes painful joint misery.

But instead of reaching for the ibuprofen for comfort, you can get the same degree of pain relief from a platter of fish or a few capsules of fish oil. Both contain omega-3 fatty acids, a super-healing polyunsaturated fat that is a natural anti-inflammatory agent. It produces the same relief that aspirin and other NSAID drugs do, but without the health risks or adverse side effects of these drugs.

HOW OMEGA-3S CALM JOINT INFLAMMATION

Researchers at the Connective Tissue Biology Laboratories in the UK have demonstrated that omega-3s silence inflammatory cytokines (the bad guys responsible for inflammation). Omega-3s also calm joint pain by boosting the body's production of anti-inflammatory fats called *resolvins*, which the body creates from the *eicosapentaenoic acid* (EPA) and *docosahexaenoic acid* (DHA) in the fat of fish. This one-two punch enables omega-3 fish oil not only to relieve pain, but literally reverse arthritic conditions in some people.

Studies show that people with moderate joint deterioration from OA and RA experience less pain when they control the inflammation in their joints and in the body as a whole. And research clearly demonstrates the remarkable capacity of fish oil to achieve this effect. Eating omega-3 fish—or taking fish oil (as you began doing on Day 3)—accomplishes this by damping down the body's production of inflammation-provoking cytokines that aggravate arthritis.

Omega-3s provide almost immediate pain relief, too. Studies show that people with OA and RA who consume omega-3 fish regularly experience less inflammation and pain, with an immediate and significant reduction in joint inflammation. In one notable study, patients who received the equivalent omega-3s of a nightly salmon dinner or daily lunchtime can of sardines reduced joint tenderness and pain by a full 50% compared to those who didn't get any fish oil. And those benefits lasted for a month after the fish oil was stopped.

BEST FISH FOR ARTHRITIS SUFFERERS

Not all fish contain omega-3s. Only certain cold-water species contain high levels of it because they manufacture the fat to keep themselves warm in frigid waters. These cold-water fish varieties are the best sources of the powerful omega-3 compounds EPA and DHA…

The Top 10 Omega-3 Rich Fish:

1. Wild Pacific salmon (fresh or canned)
2. Scallops
3. Sardines
4. Anchovies
5. Tuna
6. Halibut
7. Mackerel (not King)
8. Herring
9. Rainbow trout
10. Pacific oysters

OMEGA-3 FISH TO AVOID

To reel in these anti-arthritis benefits, you should consider eating two or three servings of omega-3 fish weekly, while avoiding all farmed fish (I'll explain why tomorrow) and larger ocean varieties, which tend to be contaminated with mercury (residue generated by the acid rain created by coal emissions). High levels of mercury have been linked to brain disorders, so pregnant women, nursing mothers, young children, and women who might become pregnant should avoid swordfish, shark, and king mackerel—and limit their consumption of other large fish, including albacore tuna and large grouper. But I think this is good advice for everyone to follow. Mercury has been linked to Alzheimer's, one of the scariest medical conditions of our time. Since mercury levels accumulate in the brain and other fatty tissues in your body, it's wise to avoid these fish.

Ironically (and tragically), these healing gifts are causing the depletion of many omega-3 fish. Worldwide demand has placed them in peril due to overfishing. The Monterrey Bay Aquaria posts a "Seafood Watch" alert on their website that serves as an updated list of endangered fish. By refusing to purchase these species, you won't be contributing to the problem—and will be doing your part to help them make a comeback. To see which fish are currently on the list, go to www.montereybayaquarium.org.

Smaller fish, such as sardines and anchovies, are fine to eat. Their omega-3 content is remarkably high—and because they have a shorter lifespan, their fat doesn't accumulate mercury residues. Other good choices are domestic shrimp (stay away from Asian or Chinese imports!), mussels, oysters, Atlantic halibut, mahi-mahi (because it reproduces abundantly and grows fast) and abalone (farmed or ocean-harvested are okay).

New Zealand green-lipped mussels (*Perna canaliculus*) are another good source of omega-3s. Two clinical studies showed eating mussels produced significant improvements in people with OA and RA. These mussels are a rich source of *glucosamine,* one of the building blocks of cartilage. (More about how you can benefit from the cartilage-regenerating ability of glucosamine in a few days). Perna is also available in supplement form.

NON-FISH SOURCES OF OMEGA-3S

Sea creatures aren't the sole source of omega-3s. Another component of omega-3 is *alpha-linolenic acid* (ALA), which is found in omega-3 plant foods. When you eat ALA-rich foods, your body converts a portion of it to EPA and DHA. So if you don't like fish, you can still pack more omega-3s into your diet without it. (I'll tell you more about these omega-3 plant foods in the days ahead.)

IT'S ALL ABOUT BALANCE

As we mentioned before, it's important to maintain an appropriate balance of omega-3s and omega-6s in your diet. Omega-3 fatty acids help reduce inflammation, while most omega-6 fatty acids tend to promote it. That's because omega-6 foods are metabolized into *arachidonic acid*, which is involved in the synthesis of pro-inflammatory molecules. The proper balance between the two helps minimize symptoms and can slow the progression of arthritis.

I don't mean to sound like a broken record about this, but consuming too many omega-6 foods will wipe out the arthritis-healing effects of any omega-3s you're consuming by interfering with the inflammation-fighting abilities of EPA and DHA. Many researchers believe this lopsided imbalance is responsible for the sharply rising rates of inflammation-driven medical conditions (including arthritis) in the US and other Westernized countries—diseases which were virtually nonexistent 100 years ago. (If you've forgotten which foods are high in omega-6s, go back to the Top Ten list I gave you on Day 4 to refresh your memory.)

70

WHAT'S FOR DINNER TONIGHT? HERE ARE TWO CHOICES:

Ready to start eating your way to better joint health? In the days and weeks ahead, you're going to be adding to your knowledge of the Arthritis Healing Foods that can minimize joint pain and help them regenerate. Here are two yummy omega-3 "meals that heal" to get you started.   NOTE: If salmon or halibut is beyond your budget right now, the grilled sardine salad is a frugal superfood alternative.) For more free arthritis-healing recipes, go to www.myhealingkitchen.com.

Mighty Omega-3 Fish over Sesame Cabbage
Serves: 2
Total prep time: 10 minutes

This quick and delicious meal contains *eight* arthritis-healing ingredients! (You already know about the fish; you'll learn about the others in the days ahead.) If you want to make this Asian-influenced dish spicier, thinly slice a red chili and add it while you're stir-frying the cabbage. BONUS: With only 419 calories, this dish also helps you lose weight. (The arthritis healing ingredients in this recipe are **bolded**).

INGREDIENTS:

Fish:
2 fresh, wild-caught **salmon** or **halibut** fillets
1 tablespoon olive oil
salt and pepper
1 lemon
¼ cup water

Cabbage:
4 cups thinly sliced Napa or red cabbage
1 tablespoon **olive oil**
1 tablespoon **sesame oil**
1 tablespoon reduced-sodium tamari or soy sauce
1 tablespoon **sesame seeds**
½ cup chopped **green onion**

DIRECTIONS:

1. Coat both sides of fish with olive oil, lemon, salt, and pepper. Bake in preheated 350 degree oven until cooked all the way through—approximately 10 minutes.

2. While fish is cooking, heat large skillet or wok. Add olive oil, then cabbage, green onion, and tamari. Stir-fry until soft. Add sesame oil and sesame seeds. Serve fish over cabbage.

> **NUTRITION FACTS:** *Calories 330, Total Fat 12.7g, Sat. Fat 1.7g, Cholesterol 58.1mg, Sodium 380.7mg, Carbs 15.7g, Fiber 4.3g, Sugars 0.0g, Protein 42.7g*

Grilled Fresh Sardines over Arugula
Serves: 4
Total prep time: 12 minutes

This dish is inspired by a classic favorite from southern Italy. We've updated it with *seven* arthritis healing ingredients to please your joints, as well as your appetite. Your budget will be happy too because sardines are an inexpensive and tasty way to get high quality omega-3s without spending a small fortune at the fish market. BONUS: This meal is ideal for losing weight, too—because each serving has only 497 calories. The arthritis healing ingredients in this recipe are **bolded**).

INGREDIENTS:

12 fresh **sardines**, cleaned, head and tails left on (or use canned)
¼ cup and 3 tablespoons **olive oil**
12 **lemon** wedges
8 cups of **arugula**
1 **red onion**, thinly sliced into ringlets
2-4 tablespoon Romano cheese
¼ cup balsamic vinegar
juice of 1 **orange**
salt and pepper
1 teaspoon Dijon mustard
1 clove of **garlic**, minced

INSTRUCTIONS:

1. Rinse the sardines under cold water. Drain and blot dry with a clean towel. Pour 3 tablespoons of olive oil over top of the sardines and toss them gently to coat. Sprinkle generously with salt and pepper on both sides.

2. Preheat the grill to medium high.

3. Cook the sardines for approximately two minutes per side.

4. Whisk together the remaining olive oil, vinegar, orange juice, mustard, garlic, salt, and pepper.

5. In a large bowl, toss the greens and onion with the dressing. Serve the fish with a sprinkle of Romano cheese on top of the salad, with a lemon wedge on the side.

> **NUTRITION FACTS:** *Calories 163, Total Fat 7.5g, Sat. Fat 2.0g, Cholesterol 58.5mg, Sodium 347mg, Carbs 7.8g, Fiber 1.8g, Sugars 0.9g, Protein 12.7g*

(–)

DAY 12: SAY NO TO FARM-RAISED FISH

HURTER: **Farm-raised fish *won't* help your arthritis—and you could end up with a tapeworm or a mouthful of neurotoxins and carcinogens. Here's why…**

IF YOU'VE RECENTLY EATEN a piece of salmon sashimi or enjoyed a Sunday brunch of lox on a bagel, chances are that your meal came from a fish farm off the west coast of Canada or Chile—even if the label claimed it to be wild-caught. "So what?" you might ask. Well, here's what…

FARMED FISH CAN MAKE YOUR JOINTS HURT

Farm-raised fish often contain lower amounts of inflammation-fighting omega-3s compared to truly wild-caught fish. And even when their omega-3 content is high, their levels of pro-inflammatory omega-6 fatty acids are disproportionally increased. This is because farmed salmon are usually fed unhealthy amounts of soy pellets, which increase their content of pro-inflammatory omega-6 fats.

The bottom line is that farmed fish can actually make joint pain *worse*—and represent a serious danger to your health and our environment. For the shocking truth about the salmon industry and how to protect yourself, please read this excellent article: www.bestlifeonline.com/cms/publish/health/The-Trouble-with-Salmon.php.

HOW SALMON FARMERS TRY TO FOOL YOU

Farmed salmon are fed artificial color to make their otherwise unappealing grayish flesh appear bright orange, like that of truly wild salmon. In the wild, salmon owe their bright pink-to-orange color to the large amounts of krill and shrimp they eat, which also accounts for their high omega-3 content. Recently, some states have passed laws requiring that "color added" appear on labels of farmed salmon, so look at them closely.

But labels aren't always a guarantee. Neither are the exorbitantly high prices that trick some consumers into believing that "if it costs more, it must be the real thing." (Wild Alaskan Chinook salmon sold for $45 a pound in 2008.) In a recent nationwide sting operation, Consumer Reports found that 56% of salmon labeled "wild" in supermarkets was actually farmed.

The stunning fact is that 90% of the fresh salmon sold in the US now comes from a farm. And most of these fish farms share the same deplorable conditions of other animal feedlot operations: overcrowding, disease contamination from pollutants and over-medication with pesticides and antibiotics.

The situation is so bad that Chile, the world's second largest salmon exporter, used 718,000 pounds of antibiotics in 2008 and more than 850,000 pounds in 2007 to contain the spread of a virus that is killing millions of its fish. When consumers eat this fish, these residues contribute to the rise of antibiotic-resistant bacteria in their bodies and in our world.

WASTED PROTEIN THAT COULD FEED HUNGRY PEOPLE

And then there's the wasteful inefficiency. It takes four pounds of wild-caught small fish (anchovies and sardines) that might otherwise feed people directly—or krill, the main food supply of many whale species—to produce a single pound of farmed salmon.

Worst of all is the pollution these open-water fish farms produce. Overcrowding in salmon farms encourages infectious *salmon anemia*, a disease that kills millions of fish and leaves survivors riddled with lesions. Farmed salmon from Chile (now a major US supplier) have been found to harbor intestinal parasites, which are passed on to humans. In other words, you can pick up a tapeworm by eating gravlax, ceviche, or sushi made with Chilean farmed salmon.

Salmon farms also attract huge populations of sea lice. Offshore fish farm cages have become virtual ranches for these parasites and pass the sea lice to wild fish, driving them to extinction. One study showed that disease and parasites spread by farmed fish are reducing wild salmon and sea trout populations by more than 50% per generation.

To rid salmon farms of the lice, Canadian fish farmers (who supply nearly 40% of the US supply) spike their feed with the marine pesticide *emamectin benzoate*, a well-know neurotoxin. Because the USDA does not regularly test imported salmon for it, this means that every piece of Canadian farmed salmon in US supermarkets is contaminated with it.

SAVVY FISH SHOPPING TIPS

■ Because of these unwise practices, Atlantic and Norwegian wild salmon have already disappeared. You can be sure that any label bearing the name "Atlantic" salmon—even if it specifically states that it is "wild"—is farmed, usually coming from Chile. But most consumers don't have a clue when it comes to purchasing salmon. A recent survey found that 90% don't know that Atlantic salmon is farm-raised, with a third believing that Atlantic is the same as "wild."

■ Look for the country of origin label (COOL) on the package. Boycott salmon from Canada, Chile, and China until these ecological travesties are corrected. Question your fish supplier closely about the origin of the fish you're buying, as well as how it was raised.

■ If you can afford it, purchase truly wild Alaskan salmon known as Chinook (also called King). Sockeye is another good choice. Other good choices are Coho, chum, and pink (most of which is canned or frozen).

■ Educate your palate. You don't have to be a gourmand to tell the difference between farmed fish and wild-caught. It's pretty obvious with the first bite. Farmed salmon, for instance, has a gooey, tasteless "fatty" flavor. Its flesh also loses its fake pink color when cooked. Once your eye becomes trained, it's easy to spot the phony fish in the store. The next time you're in the supermarket, hold a piece of wild Alaskan salmon next to a piece that is labeled "farm-raised." You'll see differences.

(+)

DAY 13: OIL YOUR JOINTS DAILY

HEALER: **Olive oil is one of your joints' best friends. It's a powerful anti-inflammatory food that prevents pain and blocks the progression of OA and RA. Eat some everyday—beginning today. Here's why...**

OLIVE OIL HEALS ARTHRITIS. In fact, this golden-green elixir is one of the most healing substances you can put in your body—and certainly flavor-enhancing. In Mediterranean cultures, it perks up the taste of everything from fish and beans to salads and bread, while helping all the foods it touches to become more healing for several medical conditions.

Along with omega-3 fish, olive oil is a mainstay of The Arthritis Healing Diet™. Its healing power lies in its *polyphenols,* powerful antioxidants (also found in green tea and red wine) which neutralize the oxidative damage that free radical molecules wreak on cells and tissues, thus accelerating the aging and disease of your joints.

OLIVE OIL COOLS JOINT PAIN

It is especially beneficial for both OA and RA because it contains a compound called *oleocanthal*, which exerts strong inflammation-taming effects. Oleocanthal blocks the production of inflammatory COX-1 and COX-2 enzymes in the same way NSAIDs do. Inhibiting these enzymes decreases inflammation and joint pain. It's no coincidence that rates of OA and RA are significantly lower in Mediterranean countries—and many researchers (myself included) believe olive oil is the main reason. It is also one of nature's best sources of *oleuropein* and *hydroxytyrosol*, two antioxidants that significantly reduce other inflammatory chemicals in the body.

Research shows that 50 milliliters of olive oil (about 3 ½ tablespoons) produces the same pain-relieving effect on your joints as a 200-mg tablet of ibuprofen. That's certainly impressive, especially when you consider that using olive oil won't put you at risk for the intestinal bleeding and kidney damage that long-term NSAIDs can.

But not all olive oil has this healing effect. You'll only receive this inflammation-fighting relief from "extra virgin olive oil" (EVOO), the liquid of the first olive pressing. This makes EVOO far richer in oleocanthal than any other types of olive oil (more about the other grades in a moment). Oleocanthal is a hero when it comes to soothing your arthritis. But it is destroyed by the heat of refining processes, which is why EVOO is the most anti-inflammatory of all the olive oil grades. It's easy to detect how "healing" the olive oil you're using is because oleocanthal produces a peppery sensation in the back of your throat. The stronger the sting, the higher its anti-inflammatory properties.

Multiply its healing power. Researchers also have discovered a couple of powerful food combinations that deliver even greater anti-inflammatory relief. One is drizzling EVOO on omega-3 fish, such as wild-caught salmon. Studies have found that eating the two together magnifies the anti-inflammatory effect each possesses.

Another powerful duo. Scientists at the University of Athens Medical School in Greece found that people who ate cooked vegetables combined with olive oil had a dramatically lower probability of developing RA. In fact, people who ate the most cooked veggies and olive oil reduced their risk for RA by a most impressive 75%. Using EVOO on veggies and salads actually boosts the antioxidant strength of those vegetables, according to a study in the *British Journal of Nutrition*.

Bonus benefits for good health. In addition to its arthritis healing power, using EVOO delivers an exceptional benefit to your heart and blood pressure. In regions of the Mediterranean where people consume a lot of olives and olive oil, death rates from heart disease are 90% lower compared to the US. And EVOO offers an exceptional cancer benefit for women. Scientists analyzing the health and diet data of 9,000 women in northern Italy discovered a 34% lower risk of breast cancer in those who consumed the most olive oil and raw vegetables compared to those who consumed the least.

EVERYTHING YOU EVER WANTED TO KNOW ABOUT OLIVE OIL

Because it's so good for your joints, here's a primer on olive oil that will make you more of a connoisseur (and impress your friends)...

■ There are three grades of olive oil: extra virgin (also called "premium extra virgin"); virgin (sometimes named "fine virgin" or "semi-fine virgin"); and "pure olive oil" or "refined olive oil."

■ Extra virgin and virgin oils are made from the first pressing of the olives, which removes about 90% of the olives' liquid. "Virgin" and "pure" olive oil are refined by heat, which seriously compromises their nutritional and anti-inflammatory properties.

■ Olive oil is produced in many countries, but most of the world's supply is produced by Spain, Italy, and Greece—with France and California now becoming major players.

OLIVE OILS FROM AROUND THE WORLD

Spanish olive oil (almost half of the world's supply) is golden-yellow in color and has a fruity-to-nutty flavor.

Italian olive oil (20% of the world's olives) is typically dark green and has an herbal aroma with grassy undertones.

Greek olive oil (13%) is also green, but has a stronger flavor.

French olive oil is pale in color with a milder flavor, indicating less oleocanthal (and therefore milder anti-inflammatory properties).

Californian olive oil is lighter in color and flavor—and is only mildly anti-inflammatory.

THE CREAM OF THE CROP

The best EVOO you can buy is labeled "estate," which means it is produced using olives from a single farm. These olives are usually handpicked (unlike other methods which wait until the olives fall to the ground before pressing), then pressed and bottled immediately. If you're in the market for the best quality, look for "estate" or "hand-picked" EVOO that says it is 100% natural, unfiltered, cold-pressed, and certified pesticide-free. This oil has the lowest acidity, richest flavor, and highest oleocanthal content. It is best appreciated in salads, as a dip for bread, or drizzled on cooked vegetables. It's well suited for uncooked dishes where you can appreciate its exquisite aroma and flavor. Expect to pay top dollar for this primo product.

"Fine virgin olive oil" is less expensive than EVOO, but is near in quality and also fine when consumed fresh and uncooked.

"Virgin olive oil" is good for cooking, and has enough flavor to be enjoyed uncooked.

"Pure olive oil" is fine for cooking, but it doesn't have enough flavor or anti-inflammatory power to be consumed uncooked.

OTHER OLIVE OIL POINTERS

Buy organic. Olives are susceptible to a pest known as the olive fly, which lives inside the olive and can damage the fruit. Fungus is another persistent problem. For these reasons, many growers use pesticides, fungicides, and herbicides to protect their crops from these pests. If you'd like to avoid these chemicals, look for labels that say "USDA Certified Organic."

Older isn't better. Oil does not improve with age—in fact, it gets worse. The older olive oil becomes, the more flavor and anti-inflammatory power it loses. Olive oil is at its peak within the two or three months after its pressing. Unfortunately, few labels carry bottling dates or "use by" dates, let alone pressing dates. Studies show that after 12 months, many of the oil's healing compounds are almost completely gone.

To avoid this problem, I order my oil from The Fresh-Pressed Olive Oil Club, a quality source that investigates reserve olive oils from around the world, then flies them to customers immediately after the pressing. It's the only way to be sure your olive oil is as fresh and healing as possible. For more information, go to www.FreshPressedOliveOil.com.

Not for high heat cooking. EVOO has a low smoke point, meaning that high heat will destroy its healing benefits—although light sautéing is acceptable. The ideal way to enjoy it is "Mediterranean style," splashed on produce and cooked vegetables. Researchers have found that consuming *no more* than two tablespoons at a time produces the optimal health benefit. Enjoy those tablespoons any way you choose—in salad dressings, as a dip for whole grain bread, or as a flavorful veggie topping. "Light" or "pure" grade olive oils can be used for higher heat uses.

Store carefully. Olive oil's high monounsaturated fat content allows it to be stored longer than most other oils without going rancid—as long as it's kept properly. Purchase EVOO in opaque or dark bottles to protect this delicate oil from light, which also can reduce its healing power. Heat and air are also enemies that create free radicals through oxidation (when the oil spoils). Not only does this leave a bad taste in your mouth, but oxidation and free radicals contribute to joint and tissue damage, heart disease, and cancer. Store it in your refrigerator or a dark, cool pantry.

The ideal storage temperature is 57 degrees Fahrenheit, but a room temperature of about 70 degrees Fahrenheit will do. If your kitchen is generally warmer than that, you may want to refrigerate the oil. Refrigeration is perfect for long-term storage of olive oil, but because chilled olive oil turns solid this isn't practical for daily use. For convenience, keep a small table supply in a tightly-capped porcelain jug to keep out air and light. This way, your olive oil is instantly ready to use. Store the rest in the fridge or another cool spot.

Use smart substitutions. Be aware that, like all fats, olive oil contains 9 calories per gram – so 3 ½ tablespoons equal 400 calories. To avoid excess calories and weight gain, use EVOO in lieu of other fats, such as butter, not in addition to them.

(-)

DAY 14: SWITCH OFF THE "NIGHTSHADES"

HURTER: **Is your arthritis being caused or aggravated by one of these common arthritis "trigger foods?" Here's the easy way to tell...**

FOR SOME PEOPLE, the alkaloids in the plant family known as *Solanaceae* (commonly called the nightshade family) seem to obstruct the body's normal repair of joint collagen. Even worse, the nightshades can accelerate cartilage degeneration and inflammation. By some estimates, up to 20% of people with arthritis feel their symptoms worsen after eating only one of these nightshade plants. Here's a list…

Nightshade Plants That May Aggravate Arthritis Pain:

- Potato
- Tomato
- Eggplant
- Red and green bell peppers
- Chili peppers
- Tobacco

DR. CHILDERS' ARTHRITIS ELIMINATION DIET

Perhaps the strongest supporter of the link between the nightshades and arthritis is Norman E. Childers, Ph.D, a professor at the University of Florida. His book, *Arthritis: Childers' Diet to Stop It!,* describes how he reversed his own arthritis by eliminating nightshades from his diet. He estimates that following his example can improve your arthritis by 70%.

It's easy enough to find out. Try cutting out all nightshade foods, as well as food products made from them—including hot sauce, ketchup, and dried red pepper flakes.

Give it 30 to 60 days to judge the effects. (You might want to start in the winter when tomatoes are out of season). Keep a diary of your results so you can chart your reduction of symptoms. Once you identify your problem "trigger foods" and the symptoms they cause, it will be easy enough to avoid them.

$$\left(+ \right)$$

DAY 15: GROW NEW CARTILAGE

HEALER: Now that you've begun to halt the inflammation and deterioration in your joints, let's help your body repair your damaged cartilage—and even begin to build a new layer...

YOU'RE HALFWAY HOME! Today marks two weeks since you began living The Arthritis Healing Lifestyle. By now you should be feeling less pain, greater energy, and more enthusiasm as you move through your world with increased ease, mobility and comfort. This means it's working!

I've saved this arthritis healing "addition" for today to celebrate your progress—and to launch you into a higher level of joint healing with a supplement that helps repair your worn-out joints by triggering the growth of new cartilage...

THE WORLD'S GREATEST ARTHRITIS SUPPLEMENT

Glucosamine-chondroitin sulfate is the top-selling arthritis supplement in the world today. The reason is simple: people realize it works. It's been proven to halt the pain and discomfort of arthritis that makes life miserable for more than 50 million Americans with OA. And medical studies confirm this healing power. If you don't know about glucosamine—or aren't taking the best form or the most effective dose—today is your lucky day!

JOINT-REPAIR IN A BOTTLE

Glucosamine-chondroitin supplements have been examined in more than 300 studies—including more than twenty double-blind clinical trials in people with arthritis.

Overall, it has proven itself successful at relieving pain and improving OA symptoms in up to 95% of people who have used it. That's an impressive stat!

In 2006, the National Institute of Health (NIH) ran the largest clinical study ever conducted on glucosamine and chondroitin called the Glucosamine/Chondroitin Arthritis Intervention Trial (GAIT). They spent $14 million confirming what a lot of us have known for some time: taking the supplement produces a significant improvement in OA symptoms. In fact, studies showed that glucosamine-chondroitin stopped joint pain and inflammation better than the leading COX-2 arthritis drugs or leading NSAID medications—without any of the drugs' side effects. Study participants reported dramatic improvements from the supplement within four weeks—and the longer they took it, the better they felt.

Other studies show that glucosamine works more effectively than NSAIDs, including naproxen, ibuprofen, and acetaminophen for relieving joint inflammation and pain. In the NIH study, people taking glucosamine-chondroitin found the longer they used them, the better their results. In most cases, relief started in less than four weeks.

IT HELPS YOUR JOINTS CREATE NEW CARTILAGE

Glucosamine-chondroitin isn't a pain-reliever per se—but it *does* decrease suffering by encouraging the creation of new cartilage. This results in less bone-on-bone contact, less inflammation, and ultimately, more comfortable joints. In fact, actual before-and-after x-rays show that taking the supplement for an extended period results in a widening of joint space, indicating new cartilage growth.

Glucosamine is a molecule your body produces to stimulate the creation of *glycosaminoglycans* (GAGs), the key components of cartilage. As we get older, the body loses its ability to make GAGS in sufficient amounts, which means cartilage is not repaired as efficiently as when you were younger. Some experts say this actually triggers the beginning of OA in many people.

Chondroitin sulfate occupies the spaces in between the collagen fibers in articular cartilage and allows it to remain stiff when compressed by attracting and holding onto fluid. Being deficient in chondroitin causes cartilage to dry out and become brittle.

HOW IT "FEEDS" YOUR CARTILAGE:

Cartilage relies on the nutrients in the *synovial fluid*, which is contained by the synovial sac encasing articular joints. Cartilage repairs itself slowly because it doesn't have a direct supply of blood like other tissue. Repair nutrients must be supplied from the synovial fluid and "squeezed" into cartilage by the compression and expansion of movement. (Think of squeezing and releasing a sponge under water to get a sense of how this works. This is why physical activity is so beneficial for people with arthritis.) Increasing your intake of glucosamine-chondroitin along with staying physically active encourages optimal cartilage regeneration.

Glucosamine is made from shellfish shells, while chondroitin is extracted from animal cartilage. These raw materials contain the nutritional building blocks that make their way into the synovial fluid to help your body form new cartilage and aid in the repair of damaged joints.

A QUALITY PRODUCT IS CRUCIAL

Plenty of people with OA take glucosamine, but many fail to experience any significant improvement. There are three reasons for this...

1. You must take the active form. Glucosamine absolutely works in helping to repair damaged cartilage (hundreds of studies prove this conclusively), but only if you take the right kind. There are three forms of glucosamine: glucosamine sulfate (SO4), glucosamine hydrochloride (HCL) and N-acetyl glucosamine (NAG). Of these, glucosamine hydrochloride is considered the most effective form, followed by glucosamine sulfate. N-acetyl glucosamine (NAG) is generally worthless—so make sure you read product labels carefully.

2. You must take the proper dose. The majority of these clinical studies use glucosamine HCL at a dose of 1,500 mg. Since pure glucosamine is very unstable, manufacturers add salt to stabilize it and to improve absorption. (Usually this is done to glucosamine sulfate.) But because salt additives diminish the amount of glucosamine available in a tablet, you must take more glucosamine sulfate (usually at least 2,500 mg of salt-stabilized glucosamine sulfate) to receive the equivalent amount of the 1,500 mg of glucosamine HCL, which is the ideal therapeutic dose. (This addition of salt explains why some people see their blood pressure rise after using glucosamine sulfate products. If you have hypertension, I suggest you stick with glucosamine HCL.) You must make this adjustment because glucosamine sulfate manufactures don't do it for you. If you're not getting the proper amount of free glucosamine, your joints can't possibly receive its cartilage healing benefits. Taking more or less doesn't work nearly as well.

Another common mistake that many experts make is to advise you to divide your dose in half and take it twice daily. This is just plain wrong. Glucosamine-chondroitin should be taken once a day to provide a maximum wallop to your bloodstream (and therefore to your joints). "Time-released glucosamine" is another bogus gimmick. You actually want the glucosamine to be released as quickly as possible so it hits your bloodstream at once. That way, more of it will be delivered to your joint fluid where it can flood cartilage cells (*chondrocytes*) with a maximum concentration. Splitting your dose deprives the chondrocytes of the amount necessary to have a beneficial effect.

3. You must buy a quality product. Get ready for a big shock: it's estimated that up to 90% of all glucosamine-chondroitin supplements are of inferior quality. Independent laboratory analysis confirms this. (This means the odds that the joint product you're currently taking could be one of them are pretty high). Even when a product label claims it is "guaranteed pure" or "laboratory tested," you still could be getting ripped off. (I'll explain why in a moment).

Shoddy, worthless joint products pervade today's marketplace. This not only wastes your hard-earned money, but it deprives your joints of the healing that a legitimate product could be providing. In the meantime, your arthritis will continue to worsen, perhaps forcing you to take pain-relieving drugs, and moving you closer to a date with the surgeon.

Dr. Jason Theodosakis, author of the 2004 bestselling book, *The Arthritis Cure (St. Martin's press, 2004),* cites an independent analysis published by a leading medical journal which evaluated 15 popular glucosamine products. The results were "astounding." They revealed that almost all products tested *failed* to contain the recommended dose of glucosamine. Only *one* actually provided the required amount that its label claimed!

How can this happen? Because no government agency regulates the quality of nutritional supplements—and quite often the raw materials are imported from foreign countries far from the reach of lawsuits by jilted consumers. In the US, anyone with enough money can start a supplement company. There are no requirements and few regulations. With more than 50 million Americans now suffering from joint problems, the temptation to profit from their pain and disability (and lack of knowledge) by producing cheap, inferior supplements is enormous.

And the cheaper the raw materials they use, the greater their profits will be. Surprisingly, quality control safeguards and supplement testing/analysis cost *more* than the supplements' raw materials. So when a company chooses the very cheapest materials for its products, it's likely to ignore quality-control procedures and product testing. If you're one of the many people that maintain that "glucosamine didn't do much for me," more than likely the fault is with the quality of the products you've been using. We *know* glucosamine-chondroitin produces improvements because hundreds of studies prove it.

HOW TO TELL THE GOOD FROM THE BAD

Since supplying your joints with the correct dose of supplemental glucosamine-chondroitin may be the single most important way you can heal them, it's essential that you know how to recognize a good product from a bad one. Here are some tips from Dr. Theo…

■ **Shop for quality, not price.** We're all trying to save money these days, but the health and healing of your joints are too important to scrimp on. No matter how cheap a brand is, it's not a bargain if it doesn't help your arthritis. Unfortunately, that's usually the case for cut-rate joint products. Some contain absolutely *zero* active ingredients.

Since no government agency goes around testing if a bottle's contents coincide with its label's claims, there's almost no way for you (the consumer) to know for sure. For instance, a few years ago researchers evaluated 32 joint supplements containing chondroitin sulfate and found that only *five* contained the 1,200 mg dose that the label claimed. (A startling 84% failed!) Researchers found that the cheapest products contained the least amount, often less than 120 mg, a dose known to be ineffective.

Does this mean you should buy the most expensive supplements? No way. In this same study, the four priciest products also flunked, proving that a high price tag isn't a reliable indicator of quality, Very low cost, however, *is* a dead giveaway that a product is of inferior quality.

■ **Steer clear of store brands.** They're usually priced well below brand name supplements because they use inferior raw materials. Store brands of shampoo, laundry detergent, and paper products may be an acceptable way to stretch your dollar, but when it comes to vitamins and supplements, "you get what you pay for." And paying half-price for a product that does your joints no good not only wastes your money, but also cheats your health.

■ **Be wary of the word "complex."** When you see that word on a label it generally means that other substances have been added to the supplement. "Complex" is a red flag telling you that the manufacturer may be adding cheaper forms of glucosamine to the product, such as N-acetyl glucosamine (NAG) or other "fillers." This will certainly diminish its effectiveness.

This is especially true when you see "chondroitin complex" on the label. Since chondroitin is an expensive raw material, some companies dilute it with MSM, hydrolyzed collagen, chicken cartilage, and other substances to increase their profit. They purposely try to deceive you by *not* listing the amount of chondroitin sulfate on the label, but rather combining it in a "complex" like this... ▢▢▢▢▢

> **Chondroitin Sulfate complex: 1,200 mg**
>
> MSM
> Hydrolyzed collagen
> Chondroitin sulfate

In this instance, the supplement may only contain 100 mg of chondroitin sulfate, with the other ingredients comprising the other 1,100 mg. You pay the premium price and they take the profit, but your poor joints lose out. You could take a product like this for years in the mistaken belief that it's helping your arthritis, while your joints will continue to deteriorate. Don't let this happen to you.

■ **Topical forms don't work.** Topically applied glucosamine-chondroitin creams and gels are bunk. It's impossible for glucosamine molecules to penetrate the skin, enter the bloodstream, and then permeate your joint fluid in significant concentrations to do any good. Save your cash.

QUALITY PRODUCTS ARE YOUR BEST ASSURANCE

Time is precious when it comes to joint healing. Since cartilage is replaced very slowly—yet destroyed quickly—time (and cartilage) lost to an inferior product may be difficult to restore. That's why it's vital that you use a joint supplement that meets the standards proven by clinical research. But how can you identify such a product? Here are some criteria...

Look for the GMP seal. This signifies that the company follows Good Manufacturing Practices (GMP). These voluntary standards describe exactly how supplement manufacturers should receive and handle raw materials, produce supplements, check for safety, and track problems and consumer complaints. Quality supplement manufacturers adhere to GMPs to separate themselves from disreputable companies. Compliance is monitored and graded by third-party audits to help assure the public that the manufacturer is conforming to these guidelines. If you don't see this seal, don't buy it.

Choose independently tested products. Several independent organizations regularly test glucosamine-chondroitin products and other nutritional supplements. Some of the more reputable labs include...

Consumer Reports (www.consumerreports.org) is a non-profit, independent organization that tests and evaluates a wide range of consumer products, including nutritional supplements. A few years ago, they tested 12 brands of joint supplements and failed three. They are the only group that lists the product failures along with the passing products. (A one-year subscription to Consumer Reports gives you access to thousands of current and past evaluations. For just $12, it's a tremendous bargain—and a smart investment.) The joint supplements they failed were...

- Now Double Strength Glucosamine & Chondroitin (Now Foods)
- ArthxDS Glucosamine Chondroitin (Pecos Pharmaceuticals)
- Solgar Extra Strength Glucosamine Chondroitin Complex

Consumer Labs (www.consumerlab.com) is another independent testing organization, although it is a for-profit corporation. (A 12-month membership costs $29.95.) They test and evaluate vitamins and supplements exclusively. In a recent report on joint supplements, half (6 out of 13) of the glucosamine-chondroitin products they examined failed to meet their labels' claims. Several chondroitin-only also flunked.

Dr. Jason Theodosakis (www.drtheo.com) has run extensive independent tests on numerous joint supplements as part of his research in writing *The Arthritis Cure*. Overall, nearly 80% of the brands he examined *failed* to meet their label claims. Two of today's very best-selling brands tested extremely poorly. One product contained only 10% of the label claim for chondroitin. The only brands to meet his stringent requirements for quality and potency so far were…

- Osteo Bi-Plex® (Rexall)
- Cosamin DS (Nutramax Labs)
- TripleAex® (Nature Made)
- Dona® (glucosamine alone, Rotta Pharmaceuticals)

Dr. Theo is continually monitoring joint products, so check with his website for new pass/fail recommendations. Dr. Theo also has formulated and currently sells his own line of joint supplements, which I have found to be of excellent quality. I'm especially impressed by his Avosoy Complete product, which contains 1,500 mg of glucosamine HCL, 800 mg of chondroitin sulfate, and 300 mg of avocado-soybean unsaponifiables (ASU). This product is free of artificial colors, flavors, or preservatives, and contains no gluten, dairy, shellfish, or cow-based products. Each and every batch is quality-tested by an independent laboratory and test results are available at his website.

Other "stamps of approval" you can trust. When shopping, look for "approval" seals from these third-party organizations…

USP-DSVP—the US pharmacopoeia dietary supplement verification program

NSF —an international dietary supplements certification program

NNFA— the National Natural Foods Association, an industry group

GHSA—the Good Housekeeping Seal of Approval

OTHER CARTILAGE REGENERATING TIPS

Stay hydrated. Cartilage is almost 80% water, so to keep it fully functional you should drink plenty of water throughout the day—and more if you drink coffee, alcohol or take diuretic medications, because they tend to dehydrate you. Drinking lots of water, as well as the Arthritis Healing Beverages suggested on Day 5, can help your joints remain more resilient.

Be sure to take vitamin B3. Some people get no relief even though they take copious amounts of glucosamine-chondroitin. In some cases, it's because they're deficient in vitamin B, especially vitamin B3 (also known as niacinamide). Dr. William Kaufman was the first to discover the amazing therapeutic effects of niacinamide in the treatment of OA and impaired joint mobility. He documented hundreds of cases of patients who became more mobile and self-sufficient after niacinamide therapy. His case histories and photos show people who were unable to raise their arms above shoulder level before treatment. After several months on niacinamide, their mobility was restored. These patients also reported a decrease in joint pain and inflammation, although niacinamide is not considered an anti-inflammatory compound or a pain-reliever. Dr. Kaufman found that niacinamide's ability to trigger actual repair of the joint surfaces caused this dramatic reduction in pain and inflammation.

Vitamin B deficiency impairs joint healing. Vitamin B deficiencies are quite common these days due to the increased use of over-the-counter and prescription drugs. Proper absorption of B vitamins requires high levels of active bacterial flora in the GI tract. But

95

this activity is inhibited by antibiotics, diuretics, oral contraceptives, acid blockers, cholesterol-lowering medications, and all forms of pain-killers. These days, it's hard to find anyone over 50 who isn't taking one of these drugs on a regular basis. NOTE: All the B vitamins work in conjunction with each other. Therefore, you can expect better results if you take niacinamide along with a good multivitamin containing a broad balance of B vitamins.

Consume sufficient protein. Adequate protein is necessary for efficient joint repair. Cartilage is high in protein, and without an adequate intake of dietary protein, your body won't have the raw materials it needs to repair your joints. I recommend you eat omega-3 fish two to three times per week and have a Berry Smoothie with whey protein powder (recipe given on Day 8) for breakfast or lunch several times per week.

Moderate your activity. Don't expect your poor joints to heal if you subject them to repetitive abuse. It's crazy to continue playing tennis or running if it hurts so much that you have to take pain pills or NSAIDs afterward. That's why I gave up golf, which was my passion for years. It just wasn't worth the chronic pain and inflammation. (Cytokine agents in inflammatory fluids act like toxic acids to destroy cartilage.)

Your inflamed joints need rest in order to heal. I switched to cycling for aerobic conditioning and added yoga, tai chi, and core-strengthening exercises such as Pilates to take the load of my joints—and it's really paid off. Range-of-motion stretches can help you maintain your flexibility and mobility without breaking a sweat (more about these activities in the days ahead.) Being overweight adds stress to weight-bearing joints, so shedding some pounds—even if only a few—will boost your comfort level. This will happen naturally by following The Arthritis Healing Diet™ you're learning about.

Allergy alert. Steer clear of glucosamine-chondroitin if you have a shellfish allergy. You can locate a shellfish-free supplement—and there are also several good vegetarian brands.

(-)

DAY 16: START SNACKING SMARTER

HURTER: **Here are the 10 worst snacks for arthritis – and the best joint-healthy substitutes that will improve your comfort and condition…**

SNACKING HAS A BAD RAP—mostly because of the junky snacks people typically munch. Quite a few of today's most popular snacks aggravate arthritis and make your joints hurt.

I'm all for snacking because it's an ideal way to keep your hunger in check between meals so you don't overeat and add to the weight your joints must bear. Snacking also helps you avoid the spikes and dips in blood sugar to balance your energy levels. But that's only if you make *good* snack choices.

Those of us with arthritis need to be especially careful to make the right picks—because the wrong snacks not only cause more inflammation and pain, but they also can accelerate joint destruction.

THE 10 WORST SNACKS FOR YOUR ARTHRITIS

As a rule of thumb, avoid virtually all vending machine options. The best arthritis snacks should "keep it real" (as in real food). Because the good stuff is so hard to find, make it a habit to carry your snacks with you—to work, on airplanes, and to the gym. This way, your hunger won't force you to eat whatever's handy. Because the "handiest" snacks are usually the ones that make your joints flare up.

Stay away from sodas, fruit drinks, and anything with sugar in it because it triggers inflammation and makes you crave more sugary foods a short time later. (Remember Day 6?) Likewise, steer clear of granola bars and energy bars, which are just candy masquerading as a pseudo-health food. Other pain activators include yogurt-covered nuts or raisins, banana chips, and so-called "natural" potato chips. Even innocent-looking pretzels act just like sugar when they hit your bloodstream because they're made with refined white flour. Hello, inflammation!

SMART SNACK SUBSTITUTIONS

Instead of choosing snacks that will inflame your joints, select these substitutes that will help calm your symptoms and keep weight stable…

Instead of:	Choose:
1. Chips	Air-popped popcorn (without butter)
2. Soda pop	One-third 100% cherry or pomegranate juice, two-thirds club soda
3. Cookies	Apple slices and five walnut halves
4. Candy bar	Six prunes (or a "thumb-size" slice of artisan cheese), six almonds
5. Ice cream	Yogurt with raisins, chopped nuts and cinnamon
6. Granola bar	Peanut butter and raisins on whole-grain bread, cut into quarters
7. Cake	Handful of mixed nuts
8. Nachos	Baby potato skins with diced spinach, onion, and cheese, baked
9. Milkshake	Fruit smoothie with plain yogurt, banana, berries, and flaxseed
10. Popsicle	10 tart fresh cherries (they're low-cal and anti-inflammatory!)

PROMISE YOUR JOINTS

Starting today, promise your joints you'll make at least one of these smart snack substitutions every day. But don't limit yourself to this short list—there's a wide world of snacks available that can help heal your arthritis and control your weight.

The ideal snack combines a complex carbohydrate food with a little protein. For example, you can pair a small handful of walnuts with a piece of fresh fruit as a mid-morning snack. The fruit releases glucose slowly and evenly because of its fiber content, so you won't get a sugar rush followed by the typical letdown. The protein in the walnuts digests even more slowly, so its effect on your appetite lasts longer.

CALORIES STILL COUNT

A snack should contain no more than 100-150 calories, and you should limit yourself to two per day, equally spaced between meals. Whatever you do, stay one step ahead of your hunger because once your stomach starts growling, you're going to eat whatever's handy. Plan ahead and always carry some healthy snacks with you when you're away from home. Cut up raw carrots, celery, broccoli, or your other favorite crunchy veggies. Dried fruit and nut mixes are good too, but they require a little discipline because they're easy to overeat and contain a lot of calories. Fruit is the original snack food and it's okay to eat it throughout the day. Take a cup of your own homemade yogurt with you to work, or a tin of omega-3 sardines with gluten-free crackers. Use the list of our Top 10 Favorite 100-calorie Snacks below as a starting point and add your own smart snacks to it. (For more Arthritis Healing Snacks, visit www.myhealingkitchen.com).

Our Top 10 Favorite 100-Calorie Arthritis Snacks:

1. Two vegetable sushi rolls
2. A piece or fresh fruit with some mixed nuts.
3. Whole wheat pita bread with one tablespoon peanut butter (or two tablespoons hummus)
4. One tablespoon peanut butter with celery sticks
5. Organic yogurt, plain or flavored (6 ounces)
6. One hard-boiled egg
7. 10 almonds or walnuts
8. Sunflower or pumpkin seeds
9. One small skim-milk cafe latte or cappuccino
10. Small cup of 1% reduced-fat cottage cheese (with cinnamon for extra blood sugar control)

(+)

DAY 17: MAKE YOUR OWN JOINT SUPPLEMENT

HEALER: The one downside of glucosamine supplements is the cost. But here's a clever idea that delivers better joint healing *absolutely free…*

PREPARE TO SAVE A BUNDLE, because today you're going to learn where to find the most effective arthritis pain-relieving supplement on earth *without* forking out $20 to $40 a bottle. In fact, it can be yours without spending a cent! All it takes are a few bones from the butcher, some crustacean shells from the local fishmonger, a bunch of eggshells, and your favorite soup kettle. That's all you need to create a high-potency "arthritis broth" full of glucosamine and chondroitin, two joint-nourishing nutrients proven to soothe your chronic arthritis joint pain and improve your condition.

THE "SECRET" INGREDIENTS IN ARTHRITIS SUPPLEMENTS

Here's a shocker: Today's top-selling joint supplement is made from raw materials that can be yours for free—or at minimal cost. Glucosamine, an essential building block of cartilage, comes from the shells of crustaceans such as crab, lobster, and shrimp. And the cartilage in soup bones is a rich source of chondroitin sulfate. (Cartilage is a form of connective tissue that contains Type II collagen, a structural protein in the body.) Together, these two compounds can help your body repair its arthritis-damaged joints, while helping the cartilage you still have to absorb more water so it stays resilient and strong.

Add plenty of chicken bones. Arthritis causes the body to trigger biochemical reactions that attack the joint. Research conducted at the Department of Pharmacy Sciences at

101

Creighton University Medical Center in Omaha, provides evidence that this initial signal to attack its own joints can be inhibited. The study shows that consumption of chicken cartilage "retrains" the immune system to no longer attack the cartilage in the joint, and is an effective therapy for treating OA and RA. Laboratory studies demonstrated that the ingestion of chicken collagen deactivates certain immune cells (killer T-cells) responsible for autoimmune disease.

The eggshell secret. A study published in a recent issue of *Clinical Rheumatology* shows that a new supplement made from eggshell membrane not only reduces joint pain and stiffness, but produces noticeable relief after only ten days. In fact, the eggshell membrane produced effects *superior* to glucosamine and chondroitin. The calcium in the shells is also great for bone health. Researchers explained that the eggshell membrane contains both glycosaminoglycans and other proteins essential for maintaining healthy cartilage in the joints. So save all your eggshells—and get your friends to help out—for the day you make...

"ARTHRITIS SOUP" FOR YOUR JOINTS

Here's the recipe for your homemade arthritis healing glucosamine-chondroitin bone broth...

1. Fill a large soup pot with beef/pork knuckles, feet, back bones, and/or joint bones. Add chicken bones and carcasses. (These gelatin-rich animal parts contain the highest concentration of chondroitin.)

2. Toss in as many crustacean shells as will fit (for their glucosamine).

3. Dump in the eggshells. Vegetable scraps are great, too.

4. Splash in some lemon juice or vinegar to release the calcium and glucosamine-chondroitin from the bones and cartilage.

5. Cover with cold water and bring to a boil. Reduce heat to a simmer, cover, and let it cook on the lowest possible heat for hours, checking the water level and heat every once in a while.

6. If scum floats to the surface, skim it off with a spoon.

7. When the broth is done, strain the liquid through a colander. Chill to remove the fat. The liquid will keep in your fridge for up to four days—or freeze it to use indefinitely. Use this "arthritis broth" as stock for a variety of soups by adding veggies, beans, and herbs. Cook whole grains in this broth, too. Or you can simply sip a hot cupful to soothe and repair your joints.

An even easier method: Place all ingredients into a slow cooker and let it simmer for a couple of days on low heat. You can also oven-roast raw bones with their meat to bring out their flavor, but it's not essential. Or you can make a seafood-only broth. Slow cook until you arrive at a gelatinous brew.

MORE POTENT THAN SUPPLEMENTS

Here's another surprise: your stove-top bone broth is a more potent arthritis healer than any glucosamine-chondroitin supplement you can buy. That's because most supplements are produced by extracting glucosamine-chondroitin with harsh chemicals that weaken their potency. On the other hand, the nutrients in this bone broth are gently leached from the bones into the water during cooking. The resulting stock is rich in digestible calcium, magnesium, phosphorus, and other trace minerals as well as glucosamine-chondroitin.

Soup stock has been simmered on kitchen stovetops all over the globe for centuries. It's an economical way to get more use from the kitchen scraps we routinely discard (another reason why arthritis wasn't such a problem in the "old days" as it is today).

Arthritis now affects nearly 80% of people over 60. Some nutritional experts believe that the absence of cartilage-rich homemade soup stock from our modern diet helps explains the current spike in rates. While it certainly isn't the sole cause, the low levels of joint-protective nutrients in our modern diet, such as collagen, hyaluronic acid, chondroitin sulfate, glycosaminoglycans (GAGs), glycine, proline (which helps create collagen), and sulfur compounds—all of which are necessary for the creation and repair of damaged joint cartilage—is an important factor.

SAVING MONEY IS GOOD FOR YOUR JOINTS

It may be time to return to the frugal ways of our forefathers. With our global economy sputtering and food prices spiking higher, the old-fashioned soup pot is making a revival. Your joints and your food budget can already benefit. So dust off your largest soup pot and press it into action. Keep it slowly simmering for days as you add more joint-healing ingredients, refilling with water as it evaporates off. Remember: the longer you cook these humble scraps, the more healing they become. (For more free Arthritis Healing Recipes, visit www.myhealingkitchen.com.)

(-)

DAY 18: BEWARE OF TRANS-FATS

HURTER: **TRANS-fat may be the most pain-provoking substance you can put in your mouth. But it can be difficult to know when you're eating it because it's hiding in so many popular food items.   Here's how to spot them...**

HOORAY FOR YOU! You've been living The Arthritis Healing Lifestyle for nearly three weeks. By now, most folks who've been practicing diligently have their symptoms under control—and have slowed or halted the progression of their condition. I hope that's you. And I also hope these remedies are becoming second-nature, as you readily recognize the substances that make your symptoms better and worse.

ARTHRITIS ENEMY NUMBER ONE

Today I'm going to tell you about one of the worst substances you can put in your mouth. Trans-fats are bad news for everyone—but especially for people with arthritis. They're highly inflammatory, and are one of the main triggers of the body's inflammation response. They have no place whatsoever in The Arthritis Healing Diet™. And medical evidence proves it …

The famous Harvard Nurses Health Study found that women who eat the most foods containing trans-fats have 73% higher levels of C-reactive protein (CRP), a marker for inflammation in the bloodstream. That's almost twice as much inflammatory activity as normal. And this directly translates into more inflammation and joint pain.

WHY TRANS-FATS ARE SO BAD FOR YOUR JOINTS

Trans-fats were invented to extend the shelf life of processed foods. They start out as the cheapest omega-6 oils—often soy, corn, cottonseed, or canola—which in themselves are pro-inflammatory. Turning them into trans-fats makes them more so.

TRANS stands for the "*TRANS*-formation" that occurs during hydrogenation, which uses high temperatures to force tiny particles of nickel into the oil. This makes the oil solid at room temperature. Food manufacturers love trans-fats because they inhibit the oxidation process that causes foods to taste rancid. Unfortunately, this also creates a toxic substance that your body can't eliminate. Trans-fats actually become a permanent part of your cell membranes.

To avoid these inflammatory fats, check food labels carefully. If you see the words "hydrogenated," "partially hydrogenated," or "stearate-rich," the food contains trans-fats—and you should drop it like a hot potato. You may be surprised to discover that the most popular processed foods, including crackers, chips, snack foods, baked goods, cookies, and doughnuts are loaded with the stuff. And fast foods are among the worst offenders. Here are some other tips that your joints will appreciate...

Eat no margarine. Avoid it no matter how "healthful" the label says it is. Margarine is hydrogenated oil, period. And don't be fooled by claims of "zero trans-fats." New laws allow food labels to say they have "none," even when the food contains a half gram or less. But there's no safe amount of trans-fats because it accumulates in your body and can't be removed.

Nix fried foods. They can contain almost 50% trans-fats. They're not only bad for your joints, but they inflame your arteries and are a major cause of heart disease. Fried chicken and French fries top the list. Your appetite may crave them, but your joints and arteries will pay the price later.

Ask questions when dining out. Some communities, such as New York City, have banned trans-fats because they're so harmful. Many companies are voluntarily abandoning them. For instance, Starbucks has eliminated TRANS-fats from all baked goods it sells nationally, and it is pushing bakers to eliminate them in baked goods they carry regionally. Avoiding foods that contain trans-fats will not only help your joints, but it could save you from a heart attack or heart disease. Do yourself a favor and "can the TRANS!"

(+)

DAY 19: HEAL YOUR JOINTS TO THE MAX WITH FLAX

HEALER: **Fish aren't the only anti-inflammatory omega-3 foods. These tasty *non-fish* sources will also increase your joint comfort and mobility...**

ADD FLAXSEEDS to your new list of Arthritis Healing Foods. They may be tiny, but their arthritis-fighting properties are impressive due to their rich supply of *alpha-linoleic acid* (ALA), one of the omega-3 fatty acids that make cold-water fish such a powerful joint protector. Flaxseed, in fact, is the very best plant source of healing omega-3s. Just two tablespoons of ground flaxseed (also called flax meal), provides you with 140% of the daily recommendation for omega-3s. And this small amount is very easy to consume.

FLAXSEED BLOCKS JOINT INFLAMMATION

As you've already learned, omega-3s reduce the inflammation underlying arthritis by helping your body produce *prostaglandins*, gatekeepers of the anti-inflammatory response. Flaxseed's arthritis protection begins when your body converts ALA into potent omega-3 EPA and DHA, the same anti-inflammatories found in omega-3-rich fish like wild salmon.

In addition to these omega-3s, flaxseed delivers significant amounts of soluble fiber, another influential inflammation-fighter. Two daily tablespoons of ground flax contains the equivalent amount of fiber you'd get from a cup of cooked oatmeal! You already may know that fiber is packed with healing benefits, but in addition to its starring role in keeping your bowels regular and your blood sugar stable, it also drives down inflammation. A University of Massachusetts Medical School study found that people whose diets include at least 20 grams of daily fiber experience 63% less inflammation than those who eat less.

FLAX ALSO FENDS OFF ARTHRITIS PAIN

Several studies show that people with OA and RA whose diets are rich sources of omega-3s experience less joint pain, too. In the UK, researchers at the Connective Tissue Biology Laboratories found that omega-3s quell the action of cytokines and interleukins, both of which are responsible for the soreness and stiffness in cartilage membranes, as well as the destruction of healthy cartilage. Flaxseed's omega-3s also soothe painful, creaky joints by increasing your body's production of anti-inflammatory fats called resolvins, which are made from the DHA and EPA your body transforms from ALA. Omega-3s also drive down leukotrienes, hormones that cause inflammation and aggravate arthritis. Research confirms that people with moderate joint deterioration have less pain when they control inflammation in joints and in their body. Flaxseed helps you do just that.

"JUST THE FLAX, MA'AM"

The best way to absorb all the arthritis healing power in flaxseed is to eat seeds that have been ground into flax meal. We suggest that you purchase whole flaxseeds, keep them in a cool place (they spoil easily when exposed to air) and use an electric coffee grinder to make fresh flax meal when you need it. Grind just enough for a week and keep the flax meal tightly covered in your refrigerator or freezer. You can also purchase pre-ground flaxseed (just be sure to keep it refrigerated). To get more than the Institute of Medicine's daily recommendation for ALA, add flax meal to your cereals, smoothies, fruit, yogurt, salads, or vegetables. I eat it whenever I can because I love its nutty flavor. You can also substitute flax meal for some of the whole wheat flour when you're baking.

FLAXSEED OIL WORKS, TOO

Flaxseed oil and flaxseed oil capsules provide you with omega-3s, but they lack the fiber of ground flax. One teaspoon of oil contains a whopping 2.5 grams of omega-3s, more than twice the amount most people get through their regular diet. For arthritis stiffness and pain, take one to three tablespoons daily, drizzled on veggies, salads, or oatmeal. Or use it to make a yummy salad dressing. Flaxseed oil is delicate, so refrigerate it and never heat or cook with it.

One caution: flax in any form thins the blood, so talk to your doctor if you're taking a prescription blood-thinner, aspirin or another NSAID. Flaxseed also lowers cholesterol, so ask your doctor about taking flax if you're on a cholesterol-lowering medication. Also, because of flax's estrogenic effect, check with your physician if you've had a hormone-sensitive cancer, such as breast cancer or uterine cancer.

(-)

DAY 20: GET OFF THAT COUCH!

HURTER: When you're sore and hurting, the last thing you want to do is get moving. But "just do it!" as they say—because immobility will make your arthritis much worse. Here's why…

MOVING YOUR BODY for just ten minutes at a time will reduce joint pain, say doctors at the American College of Rheumatology. Whether you have OA or RA, they recommend you get three daily sessions of moderate physical activity workouts of at least ten minutes each. Lifting light weights, walking briskly, or performing any non-stressful physical activity has been shown to reduce pain and increase joint and muscle mobility.

Not moving, on the other hand, actually *increases* arthritis pain. That's because failing to regularly practice range-of-motion exercises decreases your flexibility and weakens the muscles, which could provide extra support by taking the pressure off damaged joints. Moving makes it all happen.

If your arthritis is so painful that it's difficult to move at all, ask your doctor to prescribe a few physical therapy (PT) sessions, in which a trained therapist passively moves your joints gently and without strain. After you work with a PT, you can locate a personal fitness trainer called a Clinical Exercise Specialist, who has special training in medical conditions like arthritis.

START SMALL FOR BIG BENEFITS

It's hard to believe that just ten minutes of activity can be so beneficial. But research confirms that moderate exercise keeps the muscles around arthritic joints strong, while decreasing bone loss. A regular stroll around the block also lubricates joint cartilage and reduces swelling, stiffness, and pain. Exercise also helps you lose weight, which takes extra pressure off your weight-bearing joints. After only one week of regular activity, you'll notice improvements in basic functional abilities such as climbing stairs, walking, and balance—even carrying pans in the kitchen.

Another important benefit: movement chases the blues. Because depression is so common among people with arthritis, physical activity is an important psychological aspect of treatment. In a major clinical trial sponsored by the National Institutes of Health, exercise is being tested as a *primary* treatment for mild depression. Early results are positive. Also, the Surgeon General reports that moderate walking is as good as aerobics for improving both mood and general health.

STEP-BY-STEP IS BEST FOR ARTHRITIS

Movement is an important part of treatment at the Johns Hopkins Arthritis Center in Baltimore, Maryland. Therapists help patients preserve and restore their range of motion in joints, maintain and/or increase flexibility around affected joints, boost muscle strength and endurance, and improve aerobic conditioning to lift mood and decrease the health risks associated with a sedentary lifestyle. The American College of Sports Medicine recommends the following steps to accomplish those goals:

1. Begin slowly and progress gradually.

2. Avoid rapid or repetitive stressful movement of affected joints.

3. Adapt physical activity to your individual needs.

FIND TEN MINUTES TO MOVE YOUR ARTHRITIC JOINTS

If you work at a desk, get up and walk around. Or climb up and down the stairs for ten minutes. You can also stand up and do ten minutes of stretching, using your desk and chair for support. With regular practice, it's easy to increase the intensity of your workout. If you enjoy being in a group, you can go to a health club, local pool, or community fitness classes. For a regimented routine, try our 10,000 Steps Walking Plan (described <u>at www.myhealingkitchen.com</u>). Whatever your strategy, the idea is to keep moving every day, whether it's gardening, vacuuming, carrying laundry down stairs, using an elliptical machine, salsa dancing, or walking the dog in the park. Remember the old adage: use it or lose it. That's especially true for arthritic joints.

TAKE TO THE WATER

One of the best ways to overcome the tendency toward immobility and to lessen joint pain is to hit the pool. "Water walking" is especially easy on the joints because the water's buoyancy takes a big load off your joints, effectively reducing your body weight by 90%. Yet, because water is 800% more dense than air, it creates a strong resistance that really strengthens your muscles as you walk, whether it's in the shallow end of the pool or the deep end, using a flotation belt. The deeper the water, the more strenuous your workout.

Water walking is so beneficial that it's the first physical activity that elite athletes use when rehabbing after an injury or surgery. Ditto for patients in European hospitals immediately following joint replacement. It's also the therapy of choice for injured racehorses. The buoyancy of water neutralizes the pressure that gravity exerts on your damaged joints and helps the surrounding muscles get strong enough to take up the slack. Bottom line? Being in the water feels so comfortable for people with arthritis that no one can use the excuse that "exercise hurts too much" anymore.

HOW TO TAKE THE PLUNGE

■ **To start.** Stand in water that's waist or chest deep. Walk just like you would on dry land, but pumping your arms more vigorously.

■ **Watch your form.** Stand upright with your shoulders back and chest lifted. Stride forward, placing your whole foot on the bottom of the pool (not just your tiptoes). Let your heel land first, followed by the ball of your foot. To avoid straining your back, engage your core muscles but tightening you stomach as you walk.

■ **Add intensity.** As you get used to the routine, up the challenge by lifting your knees higher. Let this naturally take you into a slow "water jog" for ten strides, and return to walking. (This is called "interval training.") Try walking backward and sideways to tone other muscles. And if you really want to burn a bunch of calories, wear a weight belt and/or wrist and ankle weights!

■ **Try deep water running (DWR).** A few years ago I had lower back surgery to repair a prolapsed disk. After the surgery, my OA flared up throughout my entire body and I needed a walker to get around. I never thought I'd be able to walk normally again, let alone ever play tennis. But DWR saved the day. I hit the pool every day for an hour of walking, gradually building up to running and then wearing a weight vest along with weights on my ankles and wrists. That got me strong enough to switch to a stationary recumbent bike and gradually regain my fitness and strength. Six months after surgery I was playing tennis again—and better than I had before!

WATER RUNNING BEATS LAND JOGGING

The aerobic and calorie-burning benefits of DWR can be superior to running on land (proven in clinical studies by Hoeger et al., in 1992). This is important because succumbing to immobility because your joints hurt makes gaining weight easy, while increasing your risk of cardiovascular disease. DWR — or merely water-walking — can help you reduce your body fat and keep your heart in shape.

■ **Less stress on your heart.** Water exercise is kinder to your heart, too. Studies show that the exercising heart rate in water is up to 20 beats-per-minute lower than on land (Mougios & Deligiannis, 1993).

■ **Builds muscle tone and strength.** Shallow water aerobic exercise is also a great way to build muscular strength. One study showed that women who performed shallow water aerobics exercise for just eight weeks achieved significantly greater gains in several strength compared to the land-based control group—even though no specific muscular strength exercises were incorporated into the aqua aerobics routine (Hoeger et al., 1992).

■ **Greater flexibility.** Four separate studies confirmed that aqua exercise classes bestow increased flexibility (especially in the low back and hamstring). Researchers say that the buoyant properties of water decrease joint stress, while allowing adults to gain greater range of motion in joints and muscles.

■ **Locate a class.** With all that it has going for it, isn't it time you hit the pool? Plenty of public pools and gyms now offer aqua aerobics and aqua step classes. Some people prefer having an instructor, while others find it fun to work out in a group. To find a class near you, call your local YMCA, fitness center, or Arthritis Foundation chapter.

■ **Get some gear.** You'll be amazed at the wide array of aqua exercise equipment that's available, including aqua-steppers, aqua-cycles and water workout stations. Check out www.aquatic-exercise-equipment.com for a glimpse. Shop for water shoes (I recommend them for better traction), aqua barbells, flotation belts, aqua joggers, and a mind-boggling variety of water workout DVDs on everything from Aqua Samba to Aquatic Pilates, at www.waterworkout.com. Finally, for the ultimate in aquatic exercise luxury, you must see the underwater treadmill at www.activeforever.com. Take that, arthritis!

$$\left(+ \right)$$

DAY 21: MORE YOGURT, LESS PAIN

HEALER: **Yogurt is an excellent all-around healing food, but it is especially beneficial for arthritis for a number of important reasons. Here's how...**

YOGURT'S BEEN AROUND for thousands of years, but science is just beginning to understand its remarkable healing properties. For instance, yogurt is a potent inflammation-fighter with well-documented *curative* effects for the pain and stiffness of arthritis. This is why yogurt is an important part of The Arthritis Healing Diet™. Yogurt's beneficial bacteria not only reduce inflammation; they also strengthen the entire immune system. They even improve your body's efficiency at absorbing essential nutrients, particularly calcium.

YOGURT KEEPS INFLAMMATION LEVELS LOW

A study in the *World Journal of Gastroenterology* found that the beneficial bacteria in yogurt decreases C-reactive protein (CRP) in the body, a blood marker for inflammation. Even more compelling is that researchers noted that two bacteria strains in particular—*Lactobacillus* and *Propionibacterium*—exert an especially strong effect on CRP. This means that certain bacteria in yogurt have "strain-specific" anti-inflammatory abilities, so look for yogurt that contains these two bacteria when shopping. The same study found that probiotics cause a reduction in the body's production of cytokines, body chemicals that turn on the inflammation response in joints.

YOGURT'S "CURATIVE EFFECT" ON ARTHRITIS

Israeli medical researchers induced arthritis in a laboratory and fed one group a commercially-produced live yogurt. The results were profound. They noted that *Lactobacillus* bacteria exerted "remarkable preventive and curative" effects on arthritis.

A University of Wisconsin-Madison study found that a type of fat in milk called *conjugated linoleic acid* (CLA) snuffs out the inflammatory enzymes that aggravate RA. But CLA is only found in the milk of cows and goats that graze freely in pastures. Reason? The grasses and wild herbs they eat produce CLA in their milk. So when shopping, look for dairy products labeled as "free range" and "pasture-fed" to make sure you're getting your daily dose of inflammation-fighting CLA.

"BAD" BACTERIA MAKE JOINTS HURT

Doctors have discovered that people with RA often harbor an overgrowth of harmful bacteria in their guts—and some researchers believe there's a direct causal link. Eating live-culture yogurt can restore the balance in favor of protective anti-inflammatory bacteria. Even people who are lactose intolerant (numbering 50 million Americans who lack the enzyme needed to digest the milk sugar, lactose) can benefit from eating yogurt without the typical gas and cramping that result from consuming non-fermented dairy products. This is a definite benefit, because lactose intolerance bars these folks from the diary-based calcium which contributes to strong bones and healthy joints.

One reason yogurt is such a dynamic healer is because it's a living food that's loaded with beneficial bacteria. Eating live yogurt regularly is like sending in the cavalry to reinforce the beneficial bacteria in our GI tracts. These beneficial bugs keep the "bad guy" bacteria (such as *e coli, salmonella, listeria, campylobacter,* and *clostridium perfringens*, which cause food poisoning and other health problems) from overwhelming your body and making you ill. In fact, your GI tract is home to more than 500 species of bacteria—about 100 trillion in number! Some are beneficial and others harmful to your health. That's why the live cultures of beneficial bacteria in yogurt are called *probiotics* (literally "for life"). They are waging war 24/7 against the infectious microbes and viruses that want to colonize your body, make you sick, and eventually knock you off.

THE SECRET LINK BETWEEN ARTHRITIS AND OSTEOPOROSIS

For people with arthritis—and especially those taking steroid drugs to help manage their pain and symptoms—the danger of osteoporosis is a serious concern. Since steroids accelerate this bone-thinning condition, people taking these drugs must pay close attention to their calcium intake. And ounce-for-ounce, yogurt contains more absorbable calcium than milk. Just one cup of plain non-fat yogurt provides 414 mg of calcium, which is 25% *more* than the same amount of non-fat milk. On top of that, the milk sugar in yogurt greatly improves calcium absorption. Yogurt is also a rich source of IGF-1, the body's growth factor that regulates bone formation. Bottom line? Eating yogurt regularly isn't just good for people with arthritis—it's vital for *all* of us. More than 90% of women and 70% of men will succumb to osteoporosis in their lifetimes, which makes calcium deficiency an "epidemic" you should be concerned about.

YOGURT MAKES LOSING WEIGHT EASIER, TOO

If you have arthritis, losing weight means easing the stress on your joints. According to the National Health and Nutrition Examination Survey, women who are obese have four times the risk of knee OA than women who weigh less. And for men, the risk is nearly five times greater. Every extra pound you carry can *quadruple* the load on your joints—and that can hurt. On the bright side, every pound you lose removes four pounds of pressure from your hips and knees.

Losing weight also lowers the level of inflammatory chemicals in your bloodstream, thus easing pain. That's because fat cells, especially those around your belly, secrete pro-inflammatory hormones that raise your blood levels of C-reactive protein (CRP) and makes your joints stiff and sore. According to a study published in the *International Journal of Obesity*, when obese men and women ate three six-ounce servings of fat-free yogurt daily while on a reduced-calorie diet, they lost 22% more weight and shed 80% more abdominal fat than those who ate the same number of calories, but only one serving of dairy products. The yogurt-eaters lost an impressive 61% more body fat than the non-yogurt group. That's a big return from making such a small change!

Yogurt revs-up your metabolism, too. Another study, published in the *American Journal of Clinical Nutrition*, found that eating a diet high in calcium boosts the burn-rate of body fat. Women 18 to 30 years old with normal weights were put on either a high-calcium or a low-calcium meal plan for a full year. The high-calcium women took in 1,000 mg to 1,400 mg per day from food sources, while the low-calcium group got less than 800 mg daily. Results? The high-calcium group burned fat at *20 times* the rate of the low-calcium group. This is a true testament to calcium's fat-burning power.

NOT ALL YOGURTS ARE CREATED EQUAL

Many commercial yogurt products have been pasteurized by heat, which kills the live bacteria that make yogurt so effective against arthritis. When shopping, be sure to choose yogurt with labels marked "live active cultures." In fact, read yogurt labels carefully. Some of the most beneficial bacteria to look for include *L. bulgaricus, B. bifidus, L. casei, and L. reuteri.* Steer clear of any yogurt containing sugar, artificial sweeteners, artificial coloring or fruit. Even better and cheaper: make your own. (I'll explain how in a moment.)

How much should you eat? For maximum healing and overall good health, consume at least one cup of plain fat-free or low-fat yogurt daily. For breakfast, add your own fresh fruit, a tablespoon of ground flaxseed, chopped walnuts, and a dash of cinnamon. For lunch, blend a low-cal smoothie using fresh or frozen berries, banana, and ground flaxseed or wheat germ. You can also mix yogurt into savory dressings for salads and vegetables. Or reach for yogurt as the perfect bedtime snack. For a change of pace, try Greek yogurt, which is thicker and has a richer taste (make-your-own instructions follow). You also might like to try a glass of low-fat kefir, yogurt's liquid cousin. Kefir contains its own unique varieties of beneficial bacteria, including *Lactobacillus Caucasus*, the *Acetobacter* species, and *Streptococcus*. Feel free to add a touch of cinnamon and berry juice for flavor if you like.

HOMEMADE YOGURT IN FOUR EASY STEPS

With money so tight these days, it makes sense to make your own yogurt. Besides the money you'll save, you'll be getting a much better product because you'll *know* it contains live cultures—especially the inflammation-fighting varieties.

Making homemade yogurt is extremely easy. Just make sure all the utensils and bowls are very clean because kitchen germs and microbes can interfere with the yogurt's bacteria growth. And be patient because it takes a little practice to make great homemade yogurt—but it's well worth the effort. Just follow these easy directions...

1. In a saucepan over medium heat, warm two quarts of 2% milk (you also can use milk made from milk powder or soy milk) to the point just before it boils. Remove from heat and transfer it into a non-metal bowl or glass jar and let it cool to about 110F to 120F.

2. Gently stir in one cup of plain yogurt. (It must contain a live culture, so check the label to be sure.) The health food section of some supermarkets carry live probiotic cultures, usually in a refrigerated compartment. Look for specific bacteria that fight inflammation, such as *Lactobacillus* and *Propionibacterium*. If you are using soy milk, make sure your soy yogurt starter contains live cultures.

3. Drape a kitchen towel over the bowl or cover it with plastic wrap, punching holes in it to release the moisture.

4. Set the bowl in a warm place, like next to a heater, where the air temperature will remain about 90 degrees (F) for approximately 8 hours. Your oven is an ideal place to culture yogurt. Simply pre-heat the oven to 200 degrees F and then turn it off. Place the yogurt inside the oven once the temperature reaches about 120 degrees (F). You can do this before you go to bed and the yogurt will thicken during the night as the bacteria cultures multiply. Don't disturb the yogurt while it is thickening.

If your yogurt hasn't thickened sufficiently by morning, it's probably because the temperature wasn't warm enough. You can fix this by turning your oven on to 200 degrees (F) and placing the yogurt above it (but not actually in the oven). When the yogurt is thick enough, place it in the refrigerator where it will keep for up to one week. Stay ahead of the process so your supply doesn't run out by making a new batch regularly. If you eat a lot of yogurt, resupply your stash every few days, using one cup of the last batch as your starter.

For richer, thicker Greek yogurt: To make a thicker Greek yogurt, drain the yogurt in a muslin-cloth for about two hours. Hang it over a medium size bowl to capture the probiotic-rich liquid which you can drink. Scrape the Greek yogurt from the cloth and refrigerate it for up to one week. (For more Arthritis Healing Recipes, visit www.myhealingkitchen.com.

(-)

DAY 22: GO EASY ON ANIMAL PROTEIN

HURTER: **Overdoing it with these foods can make your joints inflamed and painful. So the best strategy is moderation—and knowing *how* your favorite animal products were raised...**

ONE QUESTION I hear a lot is, "Are eggs, red meat, and dairy foods bad for arthritis? The answer is a bit complicated. In general, these foods have gotten a bad reputation from so-called "health experts" who tell you to stay away from them for a variety of reasons. Some say they are bad for your heart and arteries. Others say they are too acidic and rob your bones of calcium. Still others believe you shouldn't eat animal products at all. I say, "nonsense."

The truth is eggs, red meat, and dairy foods are healthful foods that have been eaten safely for thousands of years. However, recent medical studies show that these foods *can* cause health problems—but not because they're unhealthful by nature. Rather, the explanation lies in how they are grown and consumed in the typical Western diet.

HOW THESE FOODS BECOME TAINTED AND INFLAMMATORY

Modern agricultural practices use hormones to accelerate the growth and production of animal products. Many farmers lace animal feed with growth hormones to make livestock bulkier and to boost their output of eggs and milk. (This is similar to bodybuilders who take steroids to make their muscles grow.) But some of these hormones also fuel the growth of tumors in humans, particularly in the breasts and prostate gland.

Another reason these animal products can become problematic is because most are of extremely poor quality. Cattle, for instance, are fed corn and grain so they become

obese quickly, mostly from increased body fat. This puts more money in farmers'
pockets, but also increases the omega-6 content of the meat and milk. Eating them in
excess as we do in the typical Western diet can make arthritis worse because they contain
high levels of arachidonic acid, an omega-6 fat that can trigger joint pain and
inflammation.

Because these factors can affect people with arthritis in different ways, you may
want to experiment with cutting back on meat to see if you feel an improvement. Many
people do—and almost immediately.

HOW TO TEST YOURSELF AND SEE:

If you have OA—and that includes an astonishing 70% of people over 65 in the
US—you may want to take a tip from John McDougall, MD. He suggests that arthritis is
actually worsened by eating certain types of animal protein.

Test his theory yourself. For the next 14 days eat no dairy, eggs, or meat—or cut down
significantly. Replace them with more veggies, fruits, legumes, and beans, plus whole
grains such as oatmeal, brown rice, nuts, and seeds. Dr McDougall says you'll feel a
definite improvement in your arthritis symptoms. Is it worth a try? You have nothing to
lose but your pain, so why not?

Why vegans have less arthritis. Studies show a vegetarian diet often makes a
difference in pain levels. Eating "vegan" means consuming only those foods which don't
come from animals, thus eliminating meat, poultry, fish, eggs and dairy products such as
milk and cheese. A 2002 research study showed that after four weeks on a low-fat vegan
diet, virtually all symptoms of RA decreased significantly. Some researchers believe that
the vegan diet works because it drastically cuts the amount of animal fats, while
emphasizing omega-3s and salicylic acid (also known as *salicin*) found in vegetables.

EXTRA BONUS: YOU'LL LOSE WEIGHT

People who eat a vegan diet also lose a lot of weight without even trying, which can bring welcome relief to achy, overburdened joints. The wealth of antioxidants in the fruits and vegetables that comprise much of a vegan diet go even further: they neutralize free radicals, the rogue oxygen molecules that attack joints. Antioxidants fight many of the symptoms of arthritis.

TO TRY A VEGAN DIET:

■ **Center your diet around** vegetables, fruits, beans and legumes, nuts and seeds and gluten-free whole grains such as brown rice. In addition, drink eight glasses of water or arthritis-friendly beverages daily to help flush toxins.

■ **Do a little reading** on veganism as you begin to eliminate animal products from your diet. You may also wish to consult with a nutritionist. You'll need to be sure to get adequate vitamin B12, iron, zinc, calcium, and protein—all of which can be found in vegan foods if your pay attention to nutritional details.

■ **Take it one step at a time.** You don't have to go "whole hog" all at once. Start slowly by adding more whole foods and fresh produce, nuts, seeds, beans, and legumes to your current diet. These should comprise approximately 60%-80% or more of your day's nutrition. Remember: it's easier to add more good foods to your Arthritis Healing Diet™ than to fight your cravings for the bad ones.

THE "HAPPY MEDIUM" SOLUTION

If you can't bear the thought of life without these animal foods, that's fine. Should you not feel any improvement in your arthritis symptoms from Dr. McDougall's two-week experiment, it's okay to invite these foods back into your diet. Just be sure that the animal products you consume have been pasture-raised and organically-fed. Also make sure no hormones were used in the development. (Studies show that pasture-raised beef contains as many omega-3s as some fish).

These healthier, higher-quality products will be more expensive than conventionally raised meat, eggs and dairy products, but the premium price is justified because they are much better for your health. Besides, the higher price tag actually works in your favor because it will help to limit your consumption. Eat these foods as occasional "treats," as side dishes, or for flavoring, like people in Mediterranean and Asian cultures, instead of having large daily portions. This will be better for your overall health and weight, as well as your arthritis.

(+)

DAY 23: A BRAZIL NUT-A-DAY KEEPS PAIN AT BAY

HEALER: **Brazil nuts are outstanding arthritis healers because they're the richest source of *selenium*, a mineral that blocks pain and nourishes joint cartilage...**

SOUNDS A BIT NUTTY, but nibbling a Brazil nut or two every day is good for your arthritis. That's because this chunky nut contains more of the trace mineral *selenium* than any other food. Selenium is especially important for people with arthritis because not getting enough of this potent antioxidant actually invites more damage to our joints. Eating selenium-rich foods also helps limit free radical molecule damage, while helping to relieve arthritis symptoms.

LOW SELENIUM, MORE ARTHRITIS

Scientists studying people with RA have identified a link between low selenium blood levels and this painful autoimmune condition in which the body attacks its own joints. They've also shown that selenium's extraordinary antioxidant action mops up joint-destroying rogue molecules. Even more interesting is that researchers found that people with low blood levels of selenium had a higher rate of OA in both knees instead of just one. Researchers explain that the pain-free knees of the higher-selenium participants are due to the mineral's nourishing effect on knee cartilage.

Why do today's foods contain less selenium? The amount of selenium a food contains varies according to the soil in which it grew or the crops that the animals were fed. In areas of the world where the soil is low in this mineral, selenium deficiency is widespread—and this is reflected in the joint problems of the local population. This is especially prevalent in certain parts of Asia, where many people have a type of arthritis called Kashin-Beck disease, or "big joint disease." Here in the US, the high plains of the Dakotas and Nebraska are rich in selenium, while deficient regions include parts of the Great Lakes east to New England, and also portions of the Pacific Northwest.

Certain arthritis drugs lower the amount of selenium circulating in your body—especially the widely prescribed anti-inflammatory *glucocorticoid* (steroid) medications such as Dexamethasone and Prednisone.

Are you selenium-deficient? Telltale signs and symptoms include unexplained fatigue, white splotchy fingernails, and frequent colds and infections.

A LITTLE SELENIUM EVERY DAY KEEPS ARTHRITIS PAIN AWAY

To ensure adequate antioxidant activity against your arthritis, be sure to get about 50 micrograms (mcg) of selenium daily. One daily Brazil nut more than covers you, since it carries from 70 to 90 mcg, depending on where it was grown. For the top food sources of selenium, see the list below. Add them all to your list of Arthritis Healing Foods. (For other Arthritis Healing Foods and free recipes, visit www.myhealingkitchen.com.)

The Top 10 Selenium Foods:

1. Brazil nuts
2. Walnuts
3. Legumes and beans
4. Crimini mushrooms
5. Seafood (including tuna, shrimp, snapper, oysters and cod)
6. Pasture-raised turkey
7. Pasture-raised beef and lamb
8. Organic pasture-raised eggs
9. Oats
10. Brown rice

(-)

DAY 24: FEWER CALORIES, MORE COMFORT

HURTER: **Everyone has their reasons for wanting to lose weight, but for people with arthritis the payoff is very direct: you'll have less pain and inflammation. Here's why…**

IF YOU'VE BEEN faithfully following these tips, chances are you've already shed a few pounds without even trying. That's because many of the "arthritis hurting" foods that make your joints ache also cause obesity and overweight. The good news is that the anti-inflammatory foods in The Arthritis Healing Diet™ are naturally low in calories, so eating them reduces your pain and your weight at the same time. Today, I urge you to commit to losing even more pounds by improving your diet and increasing your physical activity.

HOW LOSING WEIGHT IMPROVES ARTHRITIS SYMPTOMS

Losing weight improves arthritis in two important ways. A study at University of California, Berkeley found an undeniable link between the levels of C-reactive protein (CRP) and obesity. (CRP is a marker in the blood for inflammation.) Scientists discovered elevated CRP levels in 50% of overweight people they studied—and a whopping 75% for those who were obese. This compares to 25% of people in the normal weight range who had high CRP. Inflammation plays a major role in RA and OA. Body fat—especially around the waistline—secretes harmful hormones that are highly inflammatory.

In addition to increasing inflammation levels, carrying around all those extra pounds burdens your already sore weight-bearing joints. When you walk, the pressure on your knees equals five to six times your weight. So losing even five to 10 pounds can make a real difference in your comfort level.

LOSE WEIGHT AND YOUR PAIN AT THE SAME TIME

The smartest and easiest way to shed pounds is to build your diet around foods that are packed with nutrients and high in volume, but naturally low in calories. These are the ones that contain the most vitamins, minerals, fiber, and antioxidants. They also provide your body with the nutritional building blocks necessary for repair and regeneration of joint tissue and cartilage. It's a "two-fer," really. You'll lose weight without hunger or deprivation—and all those extra antioxidants will protect your joints and clean up the nasty chemicals that cause inflammation.

Research shows that antioxidants in fresh veggies and fruits help lessen the pain and symptoms of arthritis—and prevent it altogether. Eat the widest possible selection of fresh produce every day, making fresh foods the bulk of your diet. Try to consume two to three servings of omega-3 rich fish such as salmon and mackerel per week. Add brown rice and legumes, including lentils and chickpeas. Use extra virgin olive oil or yogurt for dressing salads and veggies and choose fresh herbs for seasoning in place of salt.

HOW TO EAT CARB-SMART

You began reducing your intake of refined carbohydrates (I hope!) back on Day 8. Not only are these "quickie carbs" inflammatory, but they're also a major cause of obesity. Because they're refined (which removes their fiber), these foods pack a lot of calories into a small volume, which makes it easy to consume too many before the stretch receptors in your stomach send the "I'm full" signal to your brain.

Refined carbs are everywhere today; in white-flour products such as breads and coffee cakes, in processed foods such as potato chips and crackers, soft drinks, fruit juices, coffee cakes, most breakfast cereals, and in all foods that contain sugar or high fructose corn syrup (HFCS). These foods digest quickly and cause glucose levels to quickly spike and plummet, causing rapid swings in blood sugar. That's why you're hungry again so quickly, especially for more carbohydrates.

"Smart carbs," on the other hand, still retain their fiber so they digest slowly and release their sugars into your bloodstream at a steady pace to control your hunger. They also fill you up faster on fewer calories. Their high volume and low-calorie content is the perfect combination for weight loss. Smart carbs are easy to spot because they generally remain in their original form or close to it, such as those found in fruits, vegetables, beans, nuts, seeds, and whole grains. These foods are powerful disease-fighters and ideal for insulin control.

MAKE FIBER YOUR SECRET WEIGHT LOSS ALLY

The speed with which a carb breaks down depends on the amount of fiber it contains. (Fiber is what gives a food its "roughage" or volume.) In most cases, the fiber component of a food contains no calories, so it fills you up without filling you out. By making high-fiber foods the center of your diet, you'll naturally lose weight without dieting or hunger.

Experts recommend you get a minimum of 40 grams of fiber daily for optimal health. That's easy with The Arthritis Healing Diet™ because the vast majority of foods that halt your pain and inflammation are also high in fiber. If your fiber intake could use a boost, take a look at the Top 10 Fiber Foods below for selections to include every day.

The Top 10 Fiber Foods:

Work these foods into your diet, starting your day with a bowl of oatmeal or a fiber-rich fruit smoothie, both with ground flaxseed. For lunch or dinner, open and drain a can of beans or chickpeas and dress with extra virgin olive oil and vinegar. Add raw chopped veggies or apples and a small handful of nuts. You won't believe how "filling" these fiber foods can be.

1. Psyllium seeds (ground)
2. Oat bran
3. Rice bran
4. Oatmeal
5. Beans
6. Apples
7. Grapefruit
8. Strawberries

9. Broccoli
10. Ground flaxseed

KEEP MOVING TO HURT LESS—AND LOSE MORE

It may be tempting to cut back your physical activities in the hope that you'll reduce your joint pain. But just the opposite will happen. As you learned on Day 20, inactivity actually increases arthritis pain. It also makes it easy to gain weight, which won't help matters. There are plenty of non-stressful physical activities that people with arthritis can use to maintain the range of motion in joints, while controlling their weight. For an easy way to increase your daily activity without really exercising, try my 10,000 Steps Walking Plan (described at www.myhealingkitchen.com). Or go back to Day 20 and review the many "aqua options" that allow you to burn loads of calories without burdening your joints.

BEWARE OF DINING OUT

Dining in restaurants is an easy way to consume too many calories—especially if you're dining with overweight friends. Researchers from the State University of New York at Buffalo found that overweight people eat more when they dine with an overweight friend rather than with a companion of normal weight.

The study, reported in the *American Journal of Clinical Nutrition*, illustrates how easily we can be influenced by silent peer pressure. Researchers explain that overweight friends often act as "permission-givers," making it easier for us eat foods or quantities that we know we shouldn't (or normally wouldn't). Being aware of this can help you set the example by being a leader instead of following the herd.

$$(+)$$

DAY 25: POPEYE'S SECRET

HEALER: **Popeye's spinach is a true healing food for arthritis, making it a star player in The Arthritis Healing Diet™. Here's why you should be eating more of it...**

SPINACH IS RICH in *salicylic acid* (SA), the natural compound from which the pain-relieving ingredient in aspirin, *acetylsalicylic acid*, was derived. Along with blocking pain, the SA in spinach blocks chemicals in the body that trigger inflammation. Eating spinach is like taking Mother Nature's "aspirin" with all of the pain-stopping (and preventing) benefits, but with none of the risks — such as internal bleeding, damage to the kidneys, and liver dysfunction — associated with those little white tablets.

Spinach also minimizes joint inflammation because 80% of its oil is omega-3. Plant sources of omega-3s are especially beneficial because they tend to last longer in your body. While the richest source of joint-protective omega-3s are found in cold-water fish, omega-3 plants are loaded with a unique type of the healing fatty acid known as alpha-linolenic acid (ALA), which your body stores in far greater quantities than the omegas from fish.

AN ARTHRITIS SUPER-HEALER

In addition, spinach is packed with several antioxidant vitamins that neutralize free radical molecules, which can eat away joint cartilage and tissue. One cup of raw, fresh spinach contains more than 100% of the recommended daily allowance for vitamin A, about 10% of the USDA daily allowance for vitamin C, and a healthy dose of vitamin

E. These vitamins are well known for their antioxidant powers. And there's more to spinach's arthritis-fighting prowess…

■ **Loaded with antioxidants.** Other arthritis-fighting compounds in spinach's arsenal include carotenoids and a massive dose of beta-carotene, which has been found to lower the risk of RA and other inflammatory conditions. Each of these antioxidants minimizes free radical damage that usually accelerates joint inflammation.

■ **Brimming with vitamin K.** According to a study published in *Arthritis and Rheumatism*, increasing your intake of vitamin K—which spinach is particularly rich in —helps lower the risk of OA in hands and knees by a whopping 40%. The Arthritis Foundation reports that vitamin K boosts the action of proteins that build and strengthen cartilage and bone. It also seems to reduce the pain-triggering inflammation in joints, while enhancing the ability of cartilage to withstand wear and tear. A one-cup serving of lightly boiled spinach delivers 200% of the daily Vitamin K. Steam, sauté, or quickly boil your spinach to minimize the loss of vitamin K and crank up your body's ability to absorb this essential vitamin.

■ **Chock-full of copper.** Copper is as good as gold for arthritis. This trace mineral delivers a triple dose of benefits against arthritis. It possesses an anti-inflammatory element that is vital for strong bones and healthy connective tissue. It also guards your joints against free radicals. A cup of spinach delivers 16% of your daily requirement of copper. And the reasons for eating spinach don't stop here…

HOW STRONG BONES DISCOURAGE ARTHRITIS

Spinach is also an abundant source of calcium, a very arthritis-friendly mineral. In addition to inflammation and wear and tear, OA is caused by abnormal deposits of calcium (as bone spurs) and the loss of calcium from the joints (linked to porous bones and aqueous cysts). Contrary to popular thinking, these calcium deposits are not caused by excess dietary calcium, but by a *lack* of dietary calcium. This is why spinach is so beneficial, because consuming more readily-absorbable calcium helps inhibit nasty bone spurs. One cup of steamed spinach contains an impressive 244 mg of calcium.

THE SPINACH THAT HEALS ARTHRITIS BEST

Spinach that's fresh from your backyard garden, the local farmers market, or your supermarket produce section contains the greatest amount of arthritis healing nutrients. Researchers at the University of Pennsylvania found that fresh spinach left in the refrigerator too long has less antioxidant power than canned spinach. To preserve the most nutrients, store fresh spinach in the crisper drawer of your fridge—or better yet, use it right away. Cooking fresh spinach unleashes maximum healing power because many of its nutrients are bound up and unavailable until cooking releases them. But overcooking can take a hefty toll. For maximum benefits, gently steam your spinach—or lightly sauté it over low heat in a little extra virgin olive oil.

PUT GREENS ON YOUR TABLE EVERY DAY

Researchers have discovered that people with arthritis who begin to eat a Mediterranean-style diet see a reduction in their pain, inflammation, and swollen joints after just three months. The Mediterranean menu is vegetable-centric (but not vegetarian), featuring spinach and other leafy dark greens, fresh fruit, beans, legumes and grains, regular servings of omega-3-rich fish, extra virgin olive oil, and moderate amounts of red wine. The diet minimizes the consumption of red meat, refined carbohydrates (including sugary foods and refined baked goods), and polyunsaturated vegetable oils, such as corn, safflower, soybean, and canola.

The National Institute of Arthritis and Musculoskeletal and Skin Diseases reports that fish and plant foods that are rich in omega-3 are "unquestionably anti-inflammatory agents" much like aspirin and other NSAID drugs. So, lay a piece of wild-caught salmon atop a mound of steamed spinach for a joint-healing feast. Or feed your joints one of these arthritis healing meals tonight…

Arthritis- Blocking Spinach Salad with Flax and Strawberries
Serves: 4
Total prep time: 10 minutes

Build your salad on a foundation of vitamin E and zeaxanthin, which are both amazing arthritis pain-relieving foods, and you're eating your way to better joint health. The dynamic combination of a vitamin C-rich lemon vinaigrette and strawberries teamed up with the inflammation-blocking power of ground flaxseed is a yummy way to soothe and heal your joints. (Arthritis healing ingredients in this recipe are **bolded**.)

INGREDIENTS:

½ large cucumber, peeled, seeded and halved
4 cups baby **spinach** leaves
1 small **red onion**, thinly sliced
4 teaspoons ground **flaxseed** (garnish)
8 fresh **strawberries**, sliced
4 tablespoons slivered almonds
4 tablespoons fresh goat cheese (chevre)

Dressing:
Mix **extra virgin olive oil**, red wine vinegar, **lemon juice**, plus salt and pepper to taste

INSTRUCTIONS:

1. Combine spinach, flaxseed, cucumbers and onion in a bowl.

2. Combine dressing ingredients in another bowl. Whisk together and adjust seasoning to taste.

3. Toss salad with dressing and serve each individual salad with almonds, strawberries and chevre on top. Offer freshly ground pepper at the table.

CHEF'S NOTES:

You can omit the cheese if you don't care for dairy. A sweet "nut cheese" would be delicious instead. You can substitute walnuts or pine nuts for the almonds. Remember to grind your flaxseed right before serving, and always store flaxseeds in the fridge or freezer to guard their freshness.

NUTRITION FACTS: *Calories 244, Total Fat 17.2g, Sat. Fat 8.7g, Cholesterol 26.1mg, Sodium 273mg, Carbs 11.4g, Fiber 3.7g, Sugars 2.3g, Protein 13.9g*

Anti-Inflammatory Penne with Fresh Basil and Spinach
Serves: 2-3
Total prep time: 30 minutes

This is a lighter version of one of the more decadent Italian foods. Everyone loves a little gooey mozzarella—and this dish delivers! It also delivers anti-inflammatory omega-3's from spinach and walnuts, and is loaded with inflammation-fighting onions, garlic and basil, as well as selenium boosting crimini mushrooms. *Bellisimo!* (Arthritis healing ingredients in this recipe are **bolded**.)

INGREDIENTS:

2 tablespoons **olive oil**
1 small **onion**, sliced
1 cup of sliced **crimini mushrooms**
1 bunch of **spinach** (frozen can be substituted)
1/2 cup shredded low-fat mozzarella
1 cup non-fat milk
1 cup whole grain brown rice or whole wheat penne pasta, cooked
4 cloves of **garlic**, minced
4 tablespoons chopped fresh **basil**
2 tablespoons chopped and toasted **walnuts**
2 tablespoons parmesan cheese
pinch of nutmeg
salt and pepper to taste

INSTRUCTIONS:

1. Pre-heat oven to 400 degrees.

2. Remove your cooked pasta from the fridge so it reaches room temperature.

3. Combine the olive oil, onion, mushrooms, spinach, milk, pasta, and garlic in a baking dish. Add a pinch of nutmeg and salt and pepper.

4. Sprinkle the mozzarella on top. Cover with foil and bake in the oven for 15 minutes, or until the cheese on top is melted and everything is heated through.

5. Uncover and sprinkle the parmesan and walnuts on top. Broil for 2-3 minutes, or until brown (keep an eye on it!).

6. Serve with fresh basil on top.

> **NUTRITION FACTS:** *Calories 604, Total Fat 15.9g, Sat. Fat 5.1g, Cholesterol 26mg, Sodium 418mg, Carbs 88.9g, Fiber 6.1g, Sugars 1.1g, Protein 25.6g*

(-)

DAY 26: IS WHEAT WALLOPING YOUR JOINTS?

HURTER: It's becoming the Number One food allergy in America—and most don't even know they have it. You could be one of them because the symptoms look and feel just like arthritis...

IF YOU'RE STILL suffering from joint pain, you should look into your sensitivity to gluten because that could be at the root of your problem. Gluten is a protein found in wheat, barley, rye and a seemingly endless number of other food products made with these grains. You'll find gluten in everything from pizza crust and soy sauce to envelope glue. It's also used as a texture-enhancer and thickening agent in thousands of packaged foods.

HOW GLUTEN CAUSES JOINT PAIN

Scientists have found that people who are gluten-sensitive generally don't produce the enzymes necessary to break down wheat protein, which irritates the immune system. Sensing "foreign" gluten molecules, it unleashes cytokines and other inflammatory substances to combat the perceived threat. This reaction can also inflame your joints and make them sore.

Researchers estimate that one-in-three of us has some degree of gluten sensitivity. It's one of the most common genetic conditions in the world and tends to run in families. One theory is that gluten-sensitivity started when we humans moved from being hunter-gatherers to grain farmers. It may be that some of us never developed the internal biochemistry to process the gluten in cultivated grains. Put another way, gluten may be a completely unnatural part of the human diet to which some of us have yet to adapt.

141

GLUTEN'S RELATIONSHIP TO ARTHRITIS

One study found that as many as 66% of people with *celiac disease* (a severe form of gluten sensitivity) display symptoms of joint inflammation. In another study, people with RA who followed a gluten-free diet for 14 weeks (abstaining from wheat products during this time) felt dramatic improvements in their symptoms.

Is gluten aggravating *your* arthritis? A simple way to test its effect on your arthritis symptoms is to avoid wheat, barley, and rye (and anything made with them) for one month. You'll need to read food labels very carefully and learn the "code names" for wheat used by manufacturers of processed foods. These include semolina, spelt, matzo meal, triticale, and graham flour among others.

You'll be surprised to discover that gluten is present in most processed food products, so the easiest way to avoid it is to center your diet on whole foods, spotlighting fresh veggies and fruits, legumes such as kidney beans and chickpeas, lean meats and fish, plus nuts and seeds. (For more about a gluten sensitivity diet, read up on Celiac Disease.)

WHAT TO DO IF YOU TEST POSITIVE

If your arthritis symptoms improve by avoiding gluten, you'll know you're gluten-sensitive. I recommend you consult a physician or nutritionist who specializes in celiac disease to confirm your hunch and to assist you in creating a gluten-free diet. This is your best defense. Complications from celiac disease can be serious and include osteoporosis, since the intestine is prevented from fully absorbing calcium and other bone-building minerals. Researchers at the Karolinska Institute in Sweden found that a gluten-eliminating diet can decrease the body's levels of natural antibodies that trigger RA symptoms.

$$(+)$$

DAY 27: SQUASH YOUR ARTHRITIS PAIN

HEALER: **Pumpkins aren't just for scary Halloween jack-o'-lanterns. Eating some regularly will also frighten away your joint pain. Here's how...**

SQUASH HEALS ARTHRITIS. It's a fact. Cut open the outer shell of any of the many varieties of winter squash—or open a can of pumpkin—and you'll find a joint-healing orange pulp that's loaded with *carotenoids*, potent antioxidants that neutralize one of the underlying causes of joint degeneration. For people who already have OA or RA, carotenoids block the damaging effects of free radical molecules, which set the stage for joint inflammation and pain. For those who haven't been afflicted yet, researchers say eating carotenoid-rich foods will lower your risk of ever getting RA.

HOW SQUASH CREATES STRONGER, HEALTHIER JOINTS

Winter squash and pumpkins are loaded with tongue-twisting carotenoids like *alpha-carotene, beta-carotene, beta-cryptoxanthin,* and *zeaxanthin.* The first three nutrients are converted by our bodies into the all-important vitamin A, which is essential for a strong immune system, clear vision, healthy skin, and sturdy joints. If you suffer from OA, it's possible that vitamin deficiencies could be making your problem worse. Vitamin A deficiency has been linked to diseases such as arthritis, lupus, and diabetes. Hubbard and butternut squash supply 100% of the RDA for vitamin A in a single 3-1/2 ounce serving.

Depending on the variety, winter squash can taste as sweet as pie, distinctively nutty or delicately mild. Whatever your preference, eating this carotenoid-rich vegetable lowers the risk of developing inflammatory disorders, including RA. One study involving 25,000 people at UK's University of Manchester discovered that people eating the most foods containing beta-cryptoxanthin and zeaxanthin—such as pumpkin and winter squash—had half the risk of RA compared to those who ate the least amount. It was also discovered that people with RA had a 40% lower daily intake of beta-cryptoxanthin foods and a 20% lower intake of zeaxanthin compared to those who were arthritis-free. These findings echoed previous research showing that getting as little as 400 mcg of beta-cryptoxanthin from foods —about the amount in half a large sweet potato—was linked to lower RA risk.

"SQUASH" ARTHRITIS PAIN AND INFLAMMATION

Pumpkin and all winter squash varieties are exceptionally low in calories and brimming with fiber. With only 80 calories and six grams of fiber per cup, it's the perfect inflammation-squashing food. Dietary fiber, say researchers at the Federal Research Center for Nutrition in Germany, lowers C-reactive protein (CRP), a marker in your bloodstream that indicates the presence of inflammation. CRP levels are measured to determine the effectiveness of inflammation treatments for RA. The German scientists found that men who boosted their consumption of fiber-rich foods from two to eight servings daily drove down their CRP by more than 30%. On top of that, the reduction in CRP was primarily caused by eating carotenoid-rich foods, orange-colored vegetables and fruits including pumpkin, carrots, squash, sweet potatoes, mangos, and apricots.

THE PERFECT ANTI-ARTHRITIS FOOD

Squash and pumpkin play an important dual role in The Arthritis Healing Diet™ by helping you lose the weight *and* reducing your inflammation. Researchers at the Medical University of South Carolina found that participants who ate 28 grams of fiber daily on average were able to slash their CRP levels and lose weight at the same time. Curiously, people who weighed less saw a CRP reduction of 40%, while those who were overweight only cut their CRP levels by 10%. (This confirms the link between being overweight and higher levels of inflammation.) Winter squash is also rich in manganese and vitamin C, both of which are essential for building and repairing connective tissue and reducing inflammation in arthritic joints.

BOOST ITS PAIN-RELIEVING POWER EVEN MORE

Carotenoids are fat-soluble, meaning you need to eat a little healthy fat such as extra virgin olive oil (EVOO) or sesame oil with your squash or pumpkin to help your body absorb more of their pain-relieving benefits. One very important fat-soluble nutrient in the carotenoid family is *lutein*. Research shows that people with the highest levels of lutein in their bodies are about 70% less likely to have OA of the knee, according to the National Institute of Health. Because lutein is a powerful antioxidant, eating lutein-rich foods can help ease the pain of OA or RA by neutralizing the cartilage-damaging free radicals responsible for joint damage and inflammation.

A SUPER-FRUGAL SUPERFOOD

Carotenoid-rich foods are among the most affordable fresh foods and are easy to prepare. Canned pumpkin isn't just for holiday pies. It can be added to muffins and pancakes – or stirred into your morning oatmeal. Or you can add a dollop to plain yogurt for extra flavor and healing power. You can also spoon pumpkin into tomato sauce, soups, chili, and stews to make them more inflammation-fighting. Supermarkets often carry many varieties of winter squash including butternut, delicata, and acorn squash. Also check roadside stands and farmers markets in autumn for locally-grown varieties such as buttercup, Hubbard, Japanese kabocha, and beautiful small red-orange "pie pumpkins."

AN ARTHRITIS HEALING "FAST FOOD"

Prepare this arthritis healing "squash bowl" tonight: wash a small squash, such as acorn, kabocha, or delicata, and cut it in half. Scoop out the seeds and rub a little EVOO on the inside flesh, sprinkle with cinnamon and lay the halves flesh-side down on a lightly oiled cookie sheet. Bake at 350 to 400 degrees (F) for 40 minutes to an hour, depending on thickness—or until a knife can be inserted easily. Flip them over and sprinkle the hot squash bowls with a few drops of EVOO, raisins, walnuts, plus a bit more cinnamon and nutmeg. Make a big batch so you can re-heat the leftovers for a joint-healing lunch, snack, or dinner side dish.

Don't have time to bake? You can microwave a whole squash, such as acorn, butternut, or spaghetti squash for fast results. Simply slit the skin in a few spots and microwave for seven minutes or until tender. The squash will be very hot, so wait ten minutes before cutting it in half, scraping out seeds. Spoon out the savory orange pulp, which you can mash like potatoes. Add a splash of anti-inflammatory EVOO or sesame oil, plus garlic or diced green onions. Winter squash is also delicious cubed, steamed and served cool on top of antioxidant-rich red leaf lettuce or arugula salads greens. For other arthritis healing foods and free recipes, visit www.myhealingkitchen.com. Here's another recipe you can try.

Joint-Soothing Baked Summer Squash and Spinach with Walnut Topping
Serves: 4
Total prep time: 20 minutes

You'll be fighting inflammation, dialing back your joint pain and eating great food with this spin on a classic Italian dish. Walnuts and spinach pack this dish with high levels of omega-3s. The creamy, delicious combination of Greek yogurt, garlic, and olive oil give it a richness, without the heavy dairy component of traditional recipes. (Arthritis healing ingredients in this recipe are **bolded**.)

Ingredients:

1 lb fresh, washed **spinach**
1 **summer squash**, thinly sliced
3 tbsp **extra virgin olive oil**
1 medium **onion**, chopped
2 cloves of **garlic**, minced
½ tsp grated nutmeg
½ cup plain non-fat **Greek style yogurt**, or unsweetened **soy yogurt**
½ cup whole grain breadcrumbs
1 tsp butter
1/3 cup chopped **walnuts**
Dash of **cayenne**
Salt and pepper to taste

INSTRUCTIONS:

1. Sauté spinach, squash and garlic with one tablespoon of olive oil. Add onion.

2. Transfer everything to a baking dish. Combine with yogurt, nutmeg, salt, and pepper.

Topping:

1. In a small skillet, melt butter and sauté breadcrumbs and walnuts until well combined.

2. Pour on top of spinach and squash and broil until golden brown on top. Top with freshly-ground pepper.

> **NUTRITION FACTS:** *Calories 198, Total Fat 9.8g, Sat. Fat 1.6g, Cholesterol 2.5mg, Sodium 228mg, Carbs 19.9g, Fiber 7.9g, Sugars 3.7g, Protein 13.3g*

$$\left(+\right)$$

DAY 28: BEFRIEND BROCCOLI

HEALER: **It has a world-class reputation as a health-booster and cancer-fighter. But few people know that broccoli is one of the best healing superfoods on earth.**

NO DOUBT ABOUT IT, broccoli is one of the most therapeutic foods on the planet, offering more nutrition per calorie than any other food. Superstar of the cruciferous family of vegetables, broccoli plays an important role in The Arthritis Healing Diet™. It offers significant arthritis relief because it is loaded with anti-inflammatory and antioxidant substances, including *sulforaphane*, vitamin C, vitamin K, beta carotene, calcium, and the natural pain reliever *salicylic acid*.

HOW BROCCOLI BUSTS INFLAMMATION

Broccoli blocks inflammation with sulforaphane, a naturally-occurring sulfur compound that stimulates the immune system. At Johns Hopkins, scientists discovered that sulforaphane prevents joint pain and protects cartilage in the same way COX-2 arthritis drugs do, but without the potentially dangerous side effects. Plus, the beneficial effects last longer.

Their findings, published in *Proceedings of the National Academy of Sciences*, conclude that compounds in broccoli and other cruciferous vegetables have the ability to stop pain before it starts. Sulforaphane is activated when broccoli or broccoli sprouts are chewed. When your teeth break the cells, the chemical is formed. *Diindolylmethane* (DIM) is also produced as a consequence of chewing and digesting the veggie. Studies demonstrate DIM's ability to stimulate proteins that help regulate the immune system.

This is important news for those with RA, because the immune system is intimately involved in this inflammatory condition.

WHAT'S <u>MORE</u> HEALING THAN BROCCOLI?

Broccoli sprouts contain 50 times the sulforaphane found in the mature vegetable, endowing one ounce of sprouts with as much antioxidant power as three pounds of mature broccoli. Broccoli sprouts are so tasty even kids will eat them, so be sure to add them to salads and meals as a joint-healing garnish.

BROCCOLI IS VITAL FOR HEALTHY CARTILAGE

A cup of broccoli is loaded with 123 mg of vitamin C—twice the minimum daily requirement. Studies show that people who are low in C may be at increased risk for arthritis because it is a necessary nutrient for healthy collagen and the cartilage it creates and protects. Vitamin C is effective in healing arthritis, too. As an antioxidant, it is a front-line defense against free radical damage to joints. It also facilitates the absorption of calcium, which benefits bones and cartilage.

Broccoli is also an exceptional source of vitamin K, with one cup offering 194% of the daily recommendation. Increasing your K intake, according to a study published in *Arthritis and Rheumatism*, could help lower the risk of OA in hands and knees by a whopping 40%. The Arthritis Foundation believes vitamin K boosts the action of proteins, which build and strengthen cartilage and bone. K also seems to reduce the pain-triggering inflammation in joints, while enhancing the ability of cartilage to withstand wear and tear.

In addition to vitamins C and K, broccoli has a long list of arthritis-friendly ingredients, with calcium leading the bunch. OA is caused by both abnormal deposits of calcium in the joints (called bone spurs) and the loss of calcium from the joints. Contrary to popular thinking, calcium deposits are not caused by excess dietary calcium, but by a lack of dietary calcium. This is where calcium-rich broccoli is so beneficial. One cup contains a whopping 74 mg of calcium. Finally, the beta-carotene in broccoli also has been found to lower the risk of RA and other inflammatory conditions. Broccoli delivers a significant 1,359 mcg/cup.

SELENIUM IN BROCCOLI HALTS ARTHRITIS PAIN

Broccoli is rich in selenium, too. Researchers tracking more than 900 people found those with low selenium levels in their blood had almost double the risk of developing severe arthritis. The selenium most usable by the body is called *selenium methyl selenocysteine*— and the food richest in this compound is broccoli. (Another selenium champ is garlic.)

It also contains salicylic acid (SA), the active pain-relieving ingredient in aspirin. In fact, researchers in Scotland found that vegetarians have higher levels of SA in their bloodstreams than non-vegetarians, sometimes equal to the amount in a daily aspirin. Their research, published in the British medical journal *Lancet*, noted that getting SA from food provides anti-inflammatory benefits with absolutely none of the bleeding problems caused by aspirin. Broccoli rates high in SA, along with chili peppers, cucumber, okra, and spinach.

HOW TO MAKE BROCCOLI EVEN MORE HEALING

Cut broccoli florets into smaller pieces and slice the stems into thin pieces; then let them sit for 5 to 6 minutes before cooking. This enhances their healing properties by activating beneficial enzymes. This effect is further enhanced by vitamin C, so sprinkle sliced broccoli with a little lemon juice for added therapeutic power. Once broccoli is heated, the enzymes are inactivated. For this reason, slicing broccoli will enable the enzyme to convert some of the valuable sulfur compounds before cooking.

 For maximum nutrient absorption, eat broccoli raw or steamed *al dente*. Broccoli is delicious served raw in salads, but light cooking softens its fibrous stem, aiding digestion and increasing your body's absorption of nutrients. Enjoy it both ways, and be sure to invite broccoli's cruciferous relatives—kale, cabbage, radishes, and Brussels sprouts —to your table.

AS ALWAYS, "GO ORGANIC!"

Numerous studies reveal that organically grown fruits and vegetables contain 27% more vitamin C, 29% more iron, and 14% more phosphorus, on average. Organically grown broccoli has higher levels of all its healing plant nutrients than conventionally grown. Here's a broccoli-friendly recipe for an arthritis healing breakfast that will have your joints smiling all day long...

Joint-Happy Asian Scramble
Serves: 2-3
Total prep time: 17 minutes

This quick and tasty breakfast will set you up for joint comfort all day long. Arthritis-fighting superheroes in this recipe selenium-boosting eggs, crimini mushrooms and broccoli, plus the inflammation-taming ginger, onion and garlic. (Arthritis healing ingredients in this recipe are **bolded**.)

INGREDIENTS:

2 omega-3 eggs
4 egg whites
1 cup of **crimini mushrooms**, sliced
1 cup chopped **broccoli**
½ cup chopped fresh **cilantro**
1 teaspoon grated fresh **ginger**
2 tablespoons fresh **mint**, chopped
2 cloves of **garlic**, minced
2 green **onions**, sliced
2 tablespoons **virgin coconut oil**
1 tablespoon low-sodium tamari (or soy sauce)
1/8 teaspoon **cayenne**
2 tablespoons water
1 **lime**
salt and pepper to taste

INSTRUCTIONS:

1. Heat coconut oil, garlic, and ginger in a large skillet and sauté for 2 minutes.

2. Add broccoli and mushrooms, along with 2 tablespoons of water.

3. Sauté until mushrooms are soft and broccoli has begun to cook through, about 5 minutes.   Add tamari, eggs, cayenne and salt and pepper.

4. When eggs are just about finished, add the cilantro. Serve on a plate with mint and green onions as a garnish. Squeeze fresh lime on top just before serving.

NUTRITION FACTS: *Calories 380, Total Fat 25.7g, Sat. Fat 6.3g, Cholesterol 689mg, Sodium 573mg, Carbs 9.5g, Fiber 2.1g, Sugars 0.9g, Protein 29.7g*

(+)

DAY 29: PAIN-RELIEVING PINEAPPLE

HEALER: **Prevent and relieve your joint pains with this sweet treat from the tropics. Just make sure it's fresh or else it won't work...**

PINEAPPLE (*Ananas comosus*) is a tropical fruit native to Brazil, Bolivia, and Paraguay, and is also now propagated in the Hawaiian Islands. Generations of native people have used fresh pineapple to ease their arthritis pain, both as fruit and juice. It's so potent at reducing inflammation that many boxers drink it after fights. This unique fruit contains an enzyme called *bromelain*, one of the best-researched natural anti-inflammatory agents around.

HOW PINEAPPLE HALTS ARTHRITIS INFLAMMATION

The sulfur-based bromelain in fresh pineapple quashes inflammatory agents that trigger joint pain and cartilage degeneration. A 2006 study sited in *Clinical and Experimental Rheumatology* found that a supplement containing bromelain was effective in easing discomfort from hip arthritis. The Arthritis Foundation discovered that pineapple's bromelain produces effects comparable to NSAIDs for relieving pain and inflammation. UK researchers reviewed ten studies on OA and bromelain and found that every single one confirmed bromelain's benefits.

Bromelain is also available as a supplement, and contains a concentrated source of the enzyme, although it may not be as effective as fresh pineapple. Researchers in the Dole Nutrition Institute tested fresh pineapple against six different bromelain supplements and found the enzyme activity of the fresh pineapple to be equal to and sometimes higher than the supplements. One experiment pitted a cup of pineapple against a bromelain supplement and found more than 12 times the enzyme activity in the fruit.

OTHER ARTHRITIS HEALERS HIDDEN IN THE FRUIT

Pineapple boosts the action of other supplements that help arthritis symptoms, such as glucosamine and MSM. A higher intake level of the antioxidant vitamin C is also essential for people with arthritis—and one cup of pineapple has 94% of the recommended daily allowance (RDA) for C.

Research published in *Annals of the Rheumatic Diseases* shows that vitamin C-rich foods protect against inflammatory polyarthritis, a type of RA in which two or more joints are affected. Scientists examined nutritional data on 20,000 adults and discovered that those eating the least amount of vitamin C-rich foods had more than 300% higher risk of arthritis compared to people eating the most. Pineapple is also an excellent way to get the trace mineral manganese, which is essential for building healthy joint tissue and dense bones. One cup provides 128% of the RDA for manganese, which also assists in squelching the free radicals that can damage joint cartilage.

A BITE A DAY KEEPS INFLAMMATION AWAY

The typical dose recommended for bromelain is 80 mg to 320 mg two to three times a day, equivalent to eating a fresh pineapple daily, or drinking about four cups of its juice. Try juicing your own pineapple for a bromelain-loaded, joint-soothing beverage.

Bromelain is destroyed by heat, so eating fresh pineapple provides the best benefit. Frozen pineapple retains the active enzymes, but canned fruit and juice don't (because they're pasteurized). If the fruit needs to ripen, keep it on your kitchen counter for a couple of days. You'll know it's sweet and ready to eat when the bottom softens a bit. There are several clever pineapple-coring tools that make the job easy. Refrigerate pineapple slices or chunks so you can enjoy all week long.

ENJOY IT ON AN EMPTY STOMACH

Make pineapple your between-meal arthritis healing snack of choice. When you eat it on an empty stomach, the proteolytic enzymes go right to work on your joints. When eaten with other foods, the enzymes divert their activity to digesting it, instead of the gunk in your joints. Pineapple fruit skewers are a nutritious and fun snack. Simply alternate fresh pineapple chunks with strawberries for an extra vitamin C blast and extra joint-healing. (For more Arthritis Healing Foods, Snacks and Recipes, visit www.myhealingkitchen.com.)

(+)

DAY 30: CELEBRATE!

YOU MADE IT! Today is Graduation Day—and while there are still more arthritis healing foods, recipes, and joint strengthening exercises to discover, let me congratulate you for making it through Arthritis Healing Boot Camp.

WELCOME TO THE ARTHRITIS HEALING LIFESTYLE!

So let's celebrate your liberation from arthritic captivity with a "total arthritis healing day." That means starting the day with a joint healing breakfast. Pack up your arthritis healing lunch, snacks, and beverages so you're not tempted to eat anything that will inflame your condition. Make time for some joint strengthening physical activity. And plan to end the day with a special arthritis healing dinner.

These arthritis healing superfoods, supplements, and activities you've incorporated into your life these past 30 days will keep your bloodstream stocked with natural compounds that block inflammation, prevent pain, halt the progression of your condition, and nourish the repair of your joints. But there is one piece of the healing equation that's missing—and today we're going to add it.

THE SPIRITUAL SIDE OF HEALING

Healing ourselves isn't just about repairing the physical body. It also involves healing the emotional wounds we've experienced, correcting the less-than-healthy behaviors and habits we've developed along the way, and nurturing our spiritual side.

Healing and strengthening your spirit can take many forms—and should. When researchers studied the effects of prayer, meditation, volunteerism, friendship, having a pet, or being in a loving relationship, they discovered a positive effect on the healing process from all these activities. It doesn't seem to matter which spiritual approach you take, only that you take one. There's not enough room here to discuss them all in detail, so I'm going to focus on just one of these numerous studies. And I strongly encourage you to do just that as part of your healing.

HOW MEDITATION REDUCES ARTHRITIS PAIN

Even when you're trying your best to see the sunny side of life, sometimes the challenges of living with arthritis can cause emotional distress and depression. These are the times when having a strong spiritual practice can really see you through. For example, when researchers at the University Of Maryland School Of Medicine studied the effects of a meditation program called Mindfulness-Based Stress Reduction (MBSR) on a group of people with RA they were surprised by the outcome.

For the study, half the participants were trained in MBSR, which teaches you to focus your mind on the present moment to enhance inner peace, emotional balance, and mental clarity. MBSR also presents a positive way of relating to emotions and thoughts.

Participants who were lucky enough to receive the two-month MBSR training followed it up with a 16-week maintenance program. The rest of the group was promised they'd learn MBSR at the end of the study, in exchange for periodic check-ups while serving as the control group. All participants stayed on their standard RA medical treatments and were given psychological and physical exams at the start and at two and six months into the trial.

THE RESULTS WERE IMPRESSIVE...

Those who learned and practiced MBSR showed a 35% reduction in psychological distress, with noticeable improvements in their emotional states and depression symptoms, compared to those in the control group. (In case you're interested in learning more, MBSR programs are offered at more than 200 hospitals, medical centers, and clinics worldwide.)

HOW TO TELL IF YOUR SPIRITUAL PRACTICE IS "WORKING"

Regardless of the spiritual practice you choose, there is one sure way to tell whether it's "healing" or not. And that's if it ultimately gives you a feeling of *gratitude*.

If you've been practicing these arthritis healing tips for the past 30 days, you should be feeling the rewards in less pain and more comfort, greater mobility, a happier disposition, and a more active lifestyle. Those days of needing to pop a couple of anti-inflammatory tablets or pain-relievers should be well behind you now. Sure, you may have a bad day here and there, but for the most part you're probably leading a more normal, pain-free life. If you can recall how badly you felt 30 days ago, this is something to truly be grateful for. And when it comes to helping the healing process...

"GRATITUDE IS THE ATTITUDE"

Here's a small (but hugely important) exercise that I start my day off with. It only takes about 10 or 15 minutes, but the results usually last for the entire day. I find it especially helpful for those days when nothing seems to go right. So here are my personal…

7 Steps for Cultivating Gratitude:

1. Rise a bit earlier than you normally would. Go to a quiet spot and sit comfortably with your eyes closed. Pay attention to your breath as it naturally flows in and out and let your mind clear. Scan your body from the inside, beginning at the tips of your toes as you inhale and sense your flow of attention all the way up the top of your head as you exhale. Doing this a few times will calm and center you.

2. Invite a feeling of gratitude to overtake you with each inhalation, gradually surrendering to it. Feel grateful for the moment. For being alive. For your physical body. For the mobility you still have. For the loved ones in your life. For all the things you are still able to enjoy. And everything else in your life that you appreciate.

3. Allow a smile to form on your lips even if you have to force it at first. Keep it there as you inhale and take inventory of each aspect of your present life for which you are grateful. In a short time you should feel this smile blossoming into a delightful physical sensation of happiness that will spread throughout your body and your entire being.

4. Immersed in this joy, allow yourself to be thankful in whichever manner you're most accustomed.

5. One by one, visualize the faces of people with whom you'd like to share this feeling of joyous well-being. As each person comes into your awareness, radiate this wish for health and happiness to him or her.

6. Finally, transmit this wonderful feeling outwards to our entire world and to the universe itself. Let it pour from your heart like a beam of golden light as you repeat three times:

"May all beings be Peaceful.
May all beings be Well.
May all beings Prosper.
May all beings be Happy."

7. Gather yourself by taking a big breath your eyes. Notice your surroundings in detail. With another large inhalation and exhalation, stand up and stride into your day with a giant step, open-minded and ready to learn the lessons that life has in store for you this day.

NOW IT'S TIME FOR YOUR GRADUATION

Congratulations for being such a good "student" these past 30 days! I urge you to keep a daily journal of your activities in your symptoms as a way of staying on track. This will also help you tune into your emotions and spiritual side, so you can see how they affect your physical comfort.

Remember, this isn't the end—it's just the beginning. Science is making new discoveries about arthritis every day. There are also quite a few other arthritis healing foods—plus hundreds of yummy recipes that incorporate them. I invite you to visit our website, www.myhealingkitchen.com, to continue your "education." Please write me at jim.healthy@myhealingkitchen.com and let me know how this plan is working for you. We'd love to publish your story and tell the world about YOUR success. Now it's time to celebrate with a festive arthritis healing dinner...

Anti-Arthritis Tofu Stir-Fry
Serves: 4
Total prep time: 25 minutes

With 9 healing ingredients, this stir-fry is an inflammation-conquering powerhouse. The broccoli, cabbage and tofu alone give you an anti-inflammatory jolt of omega-3 fatty acids. The veggies and pineapple supply a barrage of arthritis healing nutrients. Keep the leftovers in the fridge for a quick snack or small meal to satisfy your hunger in an instant, while providing a nutritional boost. (Arthritis healing ingredients in this recipe are **bolded.**)

INGREDIENTS:

1 lb **tofu** cut into cubes
½ cup **pineapple**, cut into bite-sized pieces
2 cups **cabbage** of your choice, shredded
½ **onion**, roughly chopped
1 cup of **broccoli** crowns, chopped
1 tablespoon minced **garlic**
2 tablespoons minced **ginger**
2 tablespoons soy sauce
1 teaspoon sesame oil
1 teaspoon **hot chili flakes** (or to taste)
1 tablespoon coconut or peanut oil
¼ cup water

INSTRUCTIONS:

1. Put oil into a hot wok or large skillet. (Cast iron works great with this.)

2. Lay the tofu in flat. Cook for one minute and then flip.

3. Remove tofu and drain on a paper towel. Add other ingredients in this order, cooking each for one minute, stirring constantly:

Ginger
Tamari
Garlic
Hot chili flakes
Onion

Broccoli
Cabbage
Pineapple
Tofu
Water
Sesame oil

4. Serve over brown rice or quinoa

> **NUTRITION FACTS:** *Calories 183, Total Fat 15.8g, Sat. Fat 4.7g, Cholesterol 0.0mg, Sodium 483mg, Carbs 13.9g, Fiber 5.0g, Sugars 0.1g, Protein 21.9g*

6 TIPS TO REMEMBER FOR ARTHRITIS COMFORT

Best of luck to you! If you have any special needs or questions, please contact me at jim.healthy@myhealingkitchen.com. And keep these six general arthritis healing guidelines in mind...

1. Focus on real foods, such as fresh fruits, vegetables, nuts, and seeds. For protein, eat quality fish and lean meats, plus legumes such as lentils and beans. Do as much shopping in the produce section as you can because this is where many of the arthritis healing foods are found.

2. For optimal health and joint comfort, prepare these foods with small quantities of high-quality, natural oils such as coconut and sesame oils when cooking. Use extra virgin olive oil when dressing salads and veggies—it is very anti-inflammatory.

3. Limit refined "food products," including most frozen meals, boxed cereals, snacks, and sweets. These can be extremely inflammatory.

4. Eat more wholesome foods, such as canned beans, tomatoes, tuna, and sardines—as well as extra virgin olive oil and live-culture yogurt. Make sure these products have no added sugar, which will fan the flames of inflammation in your joints and back.

5. Keep moving. Becoming sedentary will only make arthritis hurt more. Find some physical activities that you really enjoy and get moving for at least 30 minutes a day.

Swim, stretch, walk, or exercise in water. The more you move, the longer you will live (and the better you'll feel).

6. Take some "me time." Stress triggers pain; relaxation eases it. No matter how frantic your daily schedule may be, make sure you budget some time just for you. And use that time to unwind and center yourself. Find a spiritual practice that nurtures your spirit and let it inspire you daily. Discover how strengthening your spirit can stimulate your healing process.

ABOUT THE AUTHORS

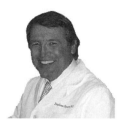

Dr. Stephen Sinatra, M.D. is a certified cardiologist, bioenergetic psychotherapist, and nutrition and anti-aging specialist with more than 20 years of experience in helping patients prevent and reverse heart disease and other chronic medical conditions. Dr. Sinatra is blazing trails and saving lives. His many books and lectures explain why inflammation is the driving force behind today's most debilitating medical conditions, including arthritis—and why food is and always has been the most powerful medicine on earth.

Dr. Sinatra is the author of the books *Lose to Win, Heartbreak and Heart Disease, Optimum Health, The CoEnzyme Q10 Phenomenon, Heart Sense for Women, Eight Weeks to Lowering Blood Pressure* and his latest books include *Spa Medicine* and *The Sinatra Solution* published by Basic Books. Dr. Sinatra also writes a monthly national newsletter entitled *Heart, Health and Nutrition*. Dr. Sinatra is a world-wide lecturer and workshop facilitator as well as being featured in several publications and medical periodicals. He is also been a featured guest on many national radio and television shows including CNN, MSNBC, and Fox on Health.

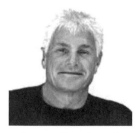

Jim Healthy™ (his pen name) is a noted health reporter and author. During his 35-year writing career, Jim has helped break the news about the biggest arthritis healing discoveries for arthritis of the past 30 years, including glucosamine-chondroitin, fish oil, omega-3 foods, and olive oil as well as the inflammatory effects of eating refined carbs and processed food products. He also writes a regular blog, www.arthritisinterrupted.com to share his discoveries about research-proven ways to halt and reverse the deterioration of arthritic joints, control pain and symptoms without drugs or painkillers, and promote the healing of damaged, worn-out cartilage.

Jim is the co-author of *The Healthy Body Book* (Penguin, 1991) and *The Fast Food Diet* with Stephen Sinatra, MD (Wiley, 2005). His most recent book is *The 30-Day Diabetes Cure* (co-authored with Dr. Stefan Ripich).

BIBLIOGRAPHY

Introduction

http://www.cdc.gov/arthritis/data_statistics.htm
http://qjmed.oxfordjournals.org/cgi/content/full/96/11/787
http://www.prolotherapy.org/prolotherapy/nsaids-bibliography
http://molecularorthopedia.com/

Day 1: Switch to Drug-Free Pain Relievers

Devil's Claw

http://rheumatology.oxfordjournals.org/cgi/content/full/41/11/1332
http://www.smart-publications.com/joint_pain/devils_claw_pain_solution.php

Boswellia

http://www.mskreport.com/articles.cfm?articleID=3107
http://www.ncbi.nlm.nih.gov/pubmed/12622457

SAM-e

http://www.biomedcentral.com/1471-2474/5/6
http://www.amjmed.com/article/0002-9343%2887%2990853-9/abstract

MSM

http://www.ncbi.nlm.nih.gov/pmc/articles/PMC2588628/
http://www.ncbi.nlm.nih.gov/pubmed/16309928

ASU

http://www.jrheum.org/content/33/8/1668.abstract
http://www.ncbi.nlm.nih.gov/pubmed/9433873

Pycnogenol

http://www.reuters.com/article/idUSCOL06848820080910
http://www.ncbi.nlm.nih.gov/pubmed/15605443

http://www.sciencedirect.com/science?_ob=ArticleURL&_udi=B6T99-4D9VFP3-3&_user=10&_coverDate=10%2F08%2F2004&_rdoc=1&_fmt=high&_orig=search&_sort=d&_docanchor=&view=c&_searchStrId=1338468525&_rerunOrigin=google&_acct=C000050221&_version=1&_urlVersion=0&_userid=10&md5=5d0c8f7b78892f8ed0bc03bafe35d3ca

Bromelain

Walker AF, et al. Bromelain reduces mild acute knee pain and improves well-being in a dose-dependent fashion in an open study of otherwise healthy adults. PHYTOMEDICINE 2002 Dec;9(8):681-6.

Klein G, Kullich W, Schnitker J, et al. Efficacy and tolerance of an oral enzyme combination in painful osteoarthritis of the hip. A double-blind, randomised study comparing oral enzymes with non-steroidal anti-inflammatory drugs. Clin Exp Rheumatol. Jan-Feb 2006;24(1):25-30.

167

Brien S, Lewith G, Walker AF, et al. Bromelain as an adjunctive treatment for moderate-to-severe osteoarthritis of the knee: a randomized placebo-controlled pilot study.QJM. Dec 2006;99(12):841-850.

Day 2: Back Off Of Painkillers

http://www.nlm.nih.gov/medlineplus/ency/article/002598.htm

http://articles.mercola.com/sites/articles/archive/2002/05/01/celebrex-vioxx-part-two.aspx

Ray W., C.Stein, K.Hall, J.Daugherty, M.Griffin. Non-steroidal anti-inflammatory drugs and risk of serious coronary heart disease: an observational cohort study. THE LANCET, Volume 359, Issue 9301, Pages 118-123.

Day 3: Get Hooked on Fish Oil

www.jrheum.org/content/33/10/1931.full.pdf
www.ncbi.nlm.nih.gov/pubmed/3030173

Day 4: Cut Back on Omega-6 Foods

http://ods.od.nih.gov/factsheets/omega3fattyacidsandhealth.asp.

Day 5: Arthritis Healing Beverages

Green Tea
www.jimmunol.org/cgi/content/abstract/170/8/4335

Ginger
www.ncbi.nlm.nih.gov/pubmed/11710709

Altman RD, Marcussen KC. Effects of a ginger extract on knee pain in patients with osteoarthritis. Arthritis Rheum. 2001;44(11):2531-2538.

Bliddal H, Rosetzsky A, Schlichting P, et al. A randomized, placebo-controlled, cross-over study of ginger extracts and ibuprofen in osteoarthritis. Osteoarthritis Cartilage. 2000;8:9-12.

Nurtjahja-Tjendraputra E, Ammit AJ, Roufogalis BD, et al. Effective anti-platelet and COX-1 enzyme inhibitors from pungent constituents of ginger. THROMB RES. 2003;111(4-5):259-265.

Thomson M, Al Qattan KK, Al Sawan SM, et al. The use of ginger (Zingiber officinale Rosc.) as a potential anti-inflammatory and antithrombotic agent. PROSTAGLANDINS LEUKOT ESSENT FATTY ACIDS. 2002;67(6):475-478.

Wigler I, Grotto I, Caspi D, et al. The effects of Zintona EC (a ginger extract) on symptomatic gonarthritis. OSTEOARTHRITIS CARTILAGE. 2003;11(11):783-789.

Pomegranate
nccam.nih.gov/research/results/spotlight/120508.htm

Cherry
jn.nutrition.org/cgi/content/full/133/6/1826

Day 6: Subtract One Soda

www.framinghamheartstudy.org/
http://www.sweetsurprise.com/experts-on-hfcs/studies

http://archpedi.ama-assn.org/cgi/content/abstract/154/6/610

Fowler, S.P. 65th Annual Scientific Sessions, American Diabetes Association, San Diego, June 10-14, 2005; Abstract 1058-P. Sharon P. Fowler, Mph, University Of Texas Health Science Center School Of Medicine, San Antonio.

Day 7: Take A Sun Bath

http://www.ncbi.nlm.nih.gov/pubmed/14730601
www.arthritis-research.com/content/10/5/R123
www.healthe-wellpc.com/pdfs/Vitamin_D_Lowering_Risk.pdf
www.ncbi.nlm.nih.gov/pubmed/14580762
www.bastyrcenter.org/content/view/749/

Day 8: Cease the Cereals

http://www.faqs.org/nutrition/Met-Obe/National-Health-and-Nutrition-Examination-Survey-NHANES.html

Day 9: Have a Berry Good Breakfast

Seymour EM, Urcuyo-Llanes D, Bolling SF, Bennink MR. Tart cherry intake reduces plasma and tissue inflammation in obesity-prone rats. FASEB Journal. 2010; 24:335.1.

Martin KR, Bopp J, Neupane S, Vega-Lopez. 100% tart cherry juice reduces plasma triglycerides and CVD risk in overweight and obese subjects. FASEB Journal. 2010; 24:722.14.

www.jacn.org/cgi/content/abstract/26/4/303
http://www.wildblueberries.com/health_benefits/research.php

Day 10: Pass on the PUFAS

www.ajcn.org/cgi/content/full/80/5/1175
www.agmrc.org/media/.../litreviewpasturemeats_96CBA3FE9B8FA.pdf
www.ncbi.nlm.nih.gov/pubmed/15329324

Day 11: Go Fishing for Healthier Joints

http://www.arthritis-relief-naturally.com/fish-oil.html

Day 12: Say No to Farm-Raised Fish

http://www.edf.org/article.cfm?contentID=5323

Day 13: Oil Your Joints Daily

www.ajcn.org/cgi/content/abstract/70/6/1077
http://journals.cambridge.org/action/displayAbstract?fromPage=online&aid=1208368
www.ncbi.nlm.nih.gov/pubmed/7927867

Day 14: Switch off the Nightshades

Childers, Norman F. Childers' Diet To Stop Arthritis: The Nightshades and Ill Health.
      Norman F. Childers Publications, 1986.

Day 15: Grow New Cartilage

www.nccam.nih.gov/research/results/gait/
Theodosakis, Jason, M.D. The Arthritis Cure. St. Martin's Press, 2004.

Day 16: Start Snacking Smarter

http://articles.mercola.com/sites/articles/archive/2010/01/19/Foods-That-Chronic-Pain-
      Sufferers-Need-to-Avoid--.aspx

Day 17: Make Your Own Joint Supplement

http://www.ncbi.nlm.nih.gov/pmc/articles/PMC2711914/

Day 18: Beware of Trans Fats

www.channing.harvard.edu/nhs/

Day 19: Heal Your Joints to the Max with Flax

www.myctm.org/articles/NP-omega-3-arthritis.php

Day 20: Get Off That Couch!

American College of Rheumatology. Exercise and Arthritis.
http://www.rheumatology.org .
http://www.ncbi.nlm.nih.gov/pubmed/17214750

Day 21: More Yogurt, Less Pain

www.wjgnet.com/1007-9327/14/5570.asp
www.ods.od.nih.gov/news/conferences/cla/cla.pdf

www.ncbi.nlm.nih.gov/pubmed/15672113
www.ars.usda.gov/pandp/people/people.htm?personid=577

Day 22: Go Easy on Animal Protein

www.pcrm.org/health/prevmed/arthritis.html

Day 23: A Brazil Nut-A-Day Keeps Pain at Bay

www.ncbi.nlm.nih.gov/pubmed/4001893

Day 24: Fewer Calories, More Comfort

www.atvb.ahajournals.org/cgi/content/short/19/4/972
www.ajcn.org/cgi/content/full/81/1/330S

Day 25: Popeye's Secret

www.health.am/ab/.../vitamin_k_deficiency_linked_to_osteoarthritis
www.ncbi.nlm.nih.gov/pubmed/12594104

Day 26: Is Wheat Walloping Your Joints?

www.celiac.com/.../1/...Gluten-Intolerance.../Page1.html
www.ajcn.org/cgi/content/full/69/3/354
www.ncbi.nlm.nih.gov/pubmed/18348715

Day 27: Squash Your Arthritis Pain

www.ncbi.nlm.nih.gov/pubmed/16087992
www.ajcn.org/cgi/content/full/84/5/1062
http://www.ncbi.nlm.nih.gov/pubmed/12578805

Day 28: Befriend Broccoli

www.brassica.com/press/pr0002.htm

Day 29: Pain Relieving Pineapple

www.ncbi.nlm.nih.gov › ... › v.1(3); Dec 2004
www.ard.bmj.com/content/4/2/43.full.pdf

Day 30: Celebrate!

www.ncbi.nlm.nih.gov/pubmed/17907231